Hepatic Encephalopathy: An Update

Guest Editors

KEVIN D. MULLEN, MD, FRCPI
RAVI K. PRAKASH, MBBS, MD, MRCP (UK)

CLINICS IN
LIVER DISEASE

www.liver.theclinics.com

Consulting Editor
NORMAN GITLIN, MD

February 2012 • Volume 16 • Number 1

SAUNDERS an imprint of ELSEVIER, Inc.

W.B. SAUNDERS COMPANY

A Division of Elsevier Inc.

1600 John F. Kennedy Boulevard, Suite 1800 ● Philadelphia, PA 19103-2899

http://www.theclinics.com

CLINICS IN LIVER DISEASE Volume 16, Number 1
February 2012 ISSN 1089-3261, ISBN-13: 978-1-4557-3885-4

Editor: Kerry Holland
Developmental Editor: Donald Mumford

Clinics in Liver Disease (ISSN 1089-3261) is published quarterly by Elsevier Inc., 360 Park Avenue South, New York, NY 10010-1710. Months of issue are February, May, August, and November. Business and Editorial Offices: 1600 John F. Kennedy Blvd., Ste. 1800, Philadelphia, PA 19103-2899. Customer Service Office: 3251 Riverport Lane, Maryland Heights, MO 63043. Periodicals postage paid at New York, NY and additional mailing offices. Subscription prices are $271.00 per year (U.S. individuals), $134.00 per year (U.S. student/resident), $365.00 per year (U.S. institutions), $360.00 per year (foreign individuals), $185.00 per year (foreign student/ resident), $440.00 per year (foreign institutions), $313.00 per year (Canadian individuals), $185.00 per year (Canadian student/resident), and $440.00 per year (Canadian institutions). Foreign air speed delivery is included in all *Clinics* subscription prices. All prices are subject to change without notice. **POSTMASTER:** Send address changes to *Clinics in Liver Disease*, Elsevier Health Sciences Division, Subscription Customer Service, 3251 Riverport Lane, Maryland Heights, MO 63043. **Customer Service: Telephone: 1-800-654-2452 (U.S. and Canada); 314-447-8871 (outside U.S. and Canada). Fax: 314-447-8029. E-mail: journalscustomer service-usa@elsevier.com (for print support); journalsonlinesupport-usa@elsevier.com (for online support).**

Reprints. For copies of 100 or more of articles in this publication, please contact the Commercial Reprints Department, Elsevier Inc., 360 Park Avenue South, New York, NY 10010-1710. Tel.: 212-633-3812; Fax: 212-462-1935; E-mail: reprints@elsevier.com.

Clinics in Liver Disease is covered in *MEDLINE/PubMed (Index Medicus)*, Science Citation Index Expanded, Journal Citation Reports/Science Edition, and Current Contents/Clinical Medicine.

Printed and bound by CPI Group (UK) Ltd, Croydon, CR0 4YY

Transferred to Digital Print 2012

Contributors

CONSULTING EDITOR

NORMAN GITLIN, MD, FRCP (LONDON), FRCPE (EDINBURGH), FACG, FACP
Formerly, Professor of Medicine, Chief of Hepatology, Emory University; Currently, Consultant, Atlanta Gastroenterology Associates, Atlanta, Georgia

GUEST EDITORS

KEVIN D. MULLEN, MD, FRCPI
Professor of Medicine, Case Western Reserve University, and Gastroenterology Division Director, MetroHealth Medical Center, Cleveland, Ohio

RAVI K. PRAKASH, MBBS, MD, MRCP (UK)
Division of Gastroenterology, MetroHealth Medical Center, Case Western Reserve University, Cleveland, Ohio

AUTHORS

JASMOHAN S. BAJAJ, MD, MSc
Associate Professor of Medicine, Division of Gastroenterology, Hepatology and Nutrition, McGuire VA Medical Center, Virginia Commonwealth University, Richmond, Virginia

FATMA BARAKAT, BA
Research Associate, SCTI Research Foundation, Coronado, California

GIAMPAOLO BIANCHI, MD
Associate Professor of Medicine, Department of Medicine and Surgery, S. Orsola-Malpighi Hospital, "Alma Mater Studiorum" University of Bologna, Bologna, Italy

SRINIVASAN DASARATHY, MD
Department of Gastroenterology and Hepatology; Department of Pathobiology, Lerner Research Institute, Cleveland Clinic, Cleveland, Ohio

R. TODD FREDERICK, MD
Division of Hepatology, Department of Transplantation, California Pacific Medical Center, San Francisco, California

MARCO GIOVAGNOLI, MD
Intern, Department of Medicine and Surgery, S. Orsola-Malpighi Hospital, "Alma Mater Studiorum" University of Bologna, Bologna, Italy

TAREK HASSANEIN, MD
Medical Director, Southern California Liver Centers; Professor, University of California, San Diego, California

ROBIN C. HILSABECK, PhD
Associate Professor, Department of Psychiatry, University of Texas Health Science Center at San Antonio; Director, Neuropsychology Postdoctoral Residency Program, South Texas Veterans Health Care System, San Antonio, Texas

E. ANTHONY JONES, MD, DSc
Fellowship Program Director, Division of Gastroenterology, MetroHealth Medical Center; Professor in Medicine, Case Western Reserve University, Cleveland, Ohio

MATTHEW R. KAPPUS, MD
Division of Gastroenterology, Hepatology and Nutrition, McGuire VA Medical Center, Virginia Commonwealth University, Richmond, Virginia

VANDANA KHUNGAR, MD, MSc
Fellow, Department of Medicine, Cedars-Sinai Medical Center; Department of Medicine, David Geffen School of Medicine at UCLA, Los Angeles, California

GIULIO MARCHESINI, MD
Professor of Medicine, Head, Unit of Metabolic Diseases and Dietetics; Intern, Department of Medicine and Surgery, S. Orsola-Malpighi Hospital, "Alma Mater Studiorum" University of Bologna, Bologna, Italy

MARK J.W. MCPHAIL, PhD, MRCP
Liver and Anti-Viral Center, Department of Medicine, St Mary's Hospital Campus, Imperial College London, London, United Kingdom

MANUELA MERLI, MD
Associate Professor of Gastroenterology, Department of Clinical Medicine, Centre for the Diagnosis and Treatment of Portal Hypertension, Sapienza University of Rome, Rome, Italy

FEDERICA MOSCUCCI, MD
Department of Clinical Medicine, Centre for the Diagnosis and Treatment of Portal Hypertension, Sapienza University of Rome, Rome, Italy

KEVIN D. MULLEN, MD, FRCPI
Professor of Medicine, Case Western Reserve University, and Gastroenterology Division Director, MetroHealth Medical Center, Cleveland, Ohio

SILVIA NARDELLI, MD
Department of Clinical Medicine, Centre for the Diagnosis and Treatment of Portal Hypertension, Sapienza University of Rome, Rome, Italy

CHIARA PASQUALE, MD
Department of Clinical Medicine, Centre for the Diagnosis and Treatment of Portal Hypertension, Sapienza University of Rome, Rome, Italy

NEERAL R. PATEL, BSc
Liver and Anti-Viral Center, Department of Medicine, St Mary's Hospital Campus, Imperial College London, London, United Kingdom

PRANAV PERIYALWAR, MD
Department of Gastroenterology, Metrohealth Medical Center; Department of Gastroenterology and Hepatology, Cleveland Clinic, Cleveland, Ohio

WILLIAM PERRY, PhD
Professor, Department of Psychiatry, Associate Director of Neuropsychiatry and
Behavioral Medicine, University of California, San Diego, San Diego, California

FRED POORDAD, MD
Chief of Hepatology and Liver Transplantation, Departments of Medicine and Surgery,
Cedars-Sinai Medical Center, Los Angeles, California

RAVI K. PRAKASH, MBBS, MD, MRCP (UK)
Division of Gastroenterology, MetroHealth Medical Center, Case Western Reserve
University, Cleveland, Ohio

LORENZO RIDOLA, MD
Department of Clinical Medicine, Centre for the Diagnosis and Treatment of Portal
Hypertension, Sapienza University of Rome, Rome, Italy

OLIVIERO RIGGIO, MD
Associate Professor of Gastroenterology, Department of Clinical Medicine, Centre for
the Diagnosis and Treatment of Portal Hypertension, Sapienza University of Rome,
Rome, Italy

MAIKO SAKAMOTO, PhD
Postdoctoral Fellow, Department of Psychiatry, University of California, San Diego,
San Diego, California

ANNA SIMONA SASDELLI, MD
Intern, Department of Medicine and Surgery, S. Orsola-Malpighi Hospital, "Alma Mater
Studiorum" University of Bologna, Bologna, Italy

SIMON D. TAYLOR-ROBINSON, MD, FRCP
Liver and Anti-Viral Center, Department of Medicine, St Mary's Hospital Campus, Imperial
College London, London, United Kingdom

Contents

The terminology of hepatic encephalopathy (HE) remained poorly defined for decades. One major problem was the lack of definition of what constituted acute versus chronic HE. Chronic HE caused more confusion because it was proposed to signify any bout of HE in patients with chronic liver disease, whereas others thought it denoted a protracted period of loss of consciousness. Numerous other versions were rampant. This mass confusion was solved by the report of the Hepatic Encephalopathy Consensus Group at the World Congress of Gastroenterology in 1998. This new multi-axial definition led to standardization of diagnosis and explosion in the field of research in HE.

The earliest hypothesis of the pathogenesis of HE implicated ammonia, although effects of appreciable concentrations of this neurotoxin did not resemble HE. Altered eurotransmission in the brain was suggested by similarities between increased GABA-mediated inhibitory neurotransmission and HE, specifically decreased consciousness and impaired motor function. Evidence of Increased GABAergic tone in models of HE has accumulated; potential mechanisms include increased synaptic availability of GABA and accumulation of natural benzodiazepine receptor ligands with agonist properties. Pathophysiological concentrations of ammonia associated with HE, have the potential of enhancing GABAergic tone by mechanisms that involve its interactions with the $GABA_A$ receptor complex.

Hepatic encephalopathy (HE) represents the effects of liver dysfunction on the brain. When HE is clinically obvious (eg, confusion, poor judgment, personality change), it is termed overt HE. The severity of HE is measured by different methods. Assessing the severity of HE is important for determining patient prognosis and effectiveness of therapy. This article discusses the different methods for grading HE, including clinical rating scales, neuropsychological tests, and neurophysiologic measures.

Minimal hepatic encephalopathy (MHE) is associated with a high risk of development of overt hepatic encephalopathy, impaired quality of life, and driving accidents. The detection of MHE requires specialized testing because it cannot, by definition, be diagnosed on standard clinical examination. Psychometric and neurophysiologic techniques are often used to test for MHE. Paper-pencil psychometric batteries and computerized tests have proved useful in diagnosing MHE and predicting its outcomes. Neurophysiologic tests also provide useful information. The diagnosis of MHE is an important issue for clinicians and patients alike. Testing strategies depend on the normative data available, patient comfort, and local expertise.

Novel imaging techniques allow the investigation of structural and functional neuropathology of hepatic encephalopathy in greater detail, but limited techniques are applicable to the clinic. Computed tomography and magnetic resonance imaging (MRI) can rule out other diagnoses and, in MRI, give diagnostic features in widely available sequences. An internationally accepted diagnostic framework that includes an objective imaging test to replace or augment psychometry remains elusive. Quantitative MRI is likely to be the best candidate to become this test. The utility of MR and nuclear medical techniques to the clinic and results from recent research are described in this article.

Hepatic encephalopathy (HE) is a potentially reversible state of impaired cognitive function or altered consciousness in patients with liver disease or portosystemic shunting. Overt HE is a particularly pressing problem. Given the many targets of treatment and lack of a clear singular cause of overt HE, there is no consensus on a single best treatment. Over the past several years, high-quality studies have been conducted on the various pharmacologic therapies for HE and, as more data emerge, hopefully HE will become a much more easily treated complication of decompensated liver disease.

Employability, driving capacity, and many domains of health-related quality of life are reduced in patients with minimal hepatic encephalopathy (HE). Moreover, once minimal HE is identified, more than 50% of patients develop overt HE within 30 months. Now that minimal HE has been shown to be associated with consequences, more studies are needed to assess the cost effectiveness to treat it. This article discusses the issues regarding diagnosis and management of minimal HE, now called "Covert HE."

Malnutrition is the most common, reversible complication of cirrhosis that adversely affects survival, response to other complications, and quality of life. Sarcopenia, or loss of skeletal muscle mass, and loss of adipose tissue and altered substrate use as a source of energy are the 2 major components of malnutrition in cirrhosis. Current therapies include high protein supplementation especially as a late evening snack. Exercise protocols have the potential of aggravating hyperammonemia and portal hypertension. Recent advances in understanding the molecular regulation of muscle mass has helped identify potential novel therapeutic targets including myostatin antagonists, and mTOR resistance.

Transjugular intrahepatic portosystemic shunt (TIPS) has been used for more than 20 years to treat some of the complications of portal hypertension. When TIPS was initially proposed, it was claimed that the optimal calibration of the shunt could allow an adequate reduction of portal hypertension, avoiding, at the same time, the occurrence of hepatic encephalopathy (HE), a neurologic syndrome. However, several clinical observations have shown that HE occurred rather frequently after TIPS, and HE has become an important issue to be taken into consideration in TIPS candidates and a problem to be faced after the procedure.

Although hepatic encephalopathy (HE) is prevalent in the cirrhotic population, it has also been considered a potentially reversible condition. Liver transplantation represents the ultimate reversal of the decompensated cirrhotic state and should provide the best option for the reversibility of HE. However, the neurologic compromise associated with HE in the cirrhotic patient may not be completely reversible. Theories regarding fixed structural and reversible metabolic deficits as well as persistence of the hyperdynamic state with continued portosystemic shunting have been proposed to explain this lack of complete reversibility. Whether this remnant neurologic deficit is clinically significant remains unclear.

The impact of overt hepatic encephalopathy on health-related quality of life is well defined, but it remains to be demonstrated how much the presence of minimal hepatic encephalopathy (MHE) might impair patients' perceived health status. MHE reduces cognitive abilities, with specific impairment in manual abilities, which can lead to a depressed mood that impairs perceived health status. Therefore, all subjects with cirrhosis should be systematically screened for MHE by validated tools. Early detection and treatment is mandatory to improve the quality of life of patients with advanced cirrhosis, their social isolation, and their daily lives.

THE CLINICS ARE NOW AVAILABLE ONLINE!

Access your subscription at:
www.theclinics.com

Preface

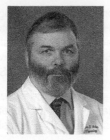 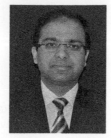

Kevin D. Mullen, MD, FRCPI   Ravi K. Prakash, MBBS, MD, MRCP (UK)
Guest Editors

The field of hepatic encephalopathy (HE) has seen major changes over the last decade. Accordingly, this is a perfect time to publish an update on this topic.

After the editors highlight some of the new perspectives on HE in the first article, Dr Jones expands on the pathogenesis of HE especially as it relates to the newer hypotheses. Dr Sakamoto and colleagues from southern California describe the assessment of HE in a very comprehensive fashion. Description of minimal HE or now-called covert HE is dealt with in great detail by Dr Kappus and Dr Bajaj from Virginia. The relatively new area on the whole spectrum of brain imaging alterations seen in patients with HE is contributed by Dr McPhail and colleagues of London, England.

The following articles describe the overall management of overt and covert HE. Dr Khungar and Dr Poordad cover the overt HE management area in detail, whereas the management of covert HE as a less developed area of therapeutics is discussed by the editors.

The article on sarcopenia or loss of lean body mass is quite unique. Lean body mass reduction is thought to modulate the expression of overt HE. Dr Periyalwar and Dr Dasarathy describe in detail our current understanding of the regulation of lean body mass in cirrhotics. Dr Riggio and colleagues in Rome have great experience in HE after the TIPS procedure and describe the current approach to this specific issue.

The last two articles in this issue touch on very important topics. These are the extent of reversibility of HE after liver transplantation and finally the relationship of HE to health-related quality of life. These articles by Todd Frederick from northern California and Giampaolo Bianchi and colleagues from Bologna, Italy finish out this update on HE.

Clin Liver Dis 16 (2012) xiii–xiv
doi:10.1016/j.cld.2012.01.002
1089-3261/12/$ – see front matter © 2012 Elsevier Inc. All rights reserved.

liver.theclinics.com

Kevin D. Mullen, MD, FRCPI
Ravi K. Prakash, MBBS, MD, MRCP (UK)

Division of Gastroenterology
MetroHealth Medical Center
Case Western Reserve University
2500 MetroHealth Drive
Cleveland, OH 44109, USA

E-mail addresses:
kevin.mullen@case.edu (K.D. Mullen)
Ravi.prakash@case.edu (R.K. Prakash)

New Perspectives in Hepatic Encephalopathy

Kevin D. Mullen, MD, FRCPI*, Ravi K. Prakash, MBBS, MD, MRCP (UK)

KEYWORDS

- Hepatic encephalopathy • Terminology • Cirrhosis
- Spectrum of neurocognitive impairment in cirrhosis

The terminology of hepatic encephalopathy (HE) remained poorly defined for decades. One major problem was the lack of definition of what constituted acute versus chronic HE.[1,2] Many physicians assumed acute HE was a term used for the fast onset of a bout of alteration in consciousness in patients with underlying cirrhosis. Others thought acute HE was the encephalopathy seen only in patients with acute liver failure. Chronic HE caused even more confusion because it was proposed by some to signify any bout of HE in patients with chronic liver disease, whereas others thought it denoted a protracted (length of time specified) period of loss of consciousness. Numerous other confusions were rampant; at times, articles were being turned down by journals because of inexact terminology when, in fact, standardized terminology had never been established.

This mass confusion was solved, to a significant extent, by the report of the Hepatic Encephalopathy Consensus Group at the World Congress of Gastroenterology in Vienna in 1998. This report led to an entirely new multiaxial definition for the terminology of HE (**Fig. 1**).

As noted, 3 broad types of HE were defined. Type A signified the HE associated with acute liver failure. Type B was designated to represent the rare form of HE associated with portosystemic bypass in the absence of any intrinsic liver disease. Finally, type C HE referred to the encephalopathy associated with chronic liver disease, which is primarily cirrhosis. Under the categories of type B and C HE, there are further terms subdividing HE into episodic HE, persistent HE and subtle form called minimal HE.

As it turned out, the recommendation of the term minimal HE, along with acceptable diagnostic criteria for this form of HE, had a major impact on the field of HE. Multiple articles have appeared using this terminology and diagnostic criteria.[3] Minimal HE is now known to be associated with the reduction in quality of life[4,5]; reduced driving skills[6–8]; reduced ability to hold certain kinds of employment[9,10]; and, most importantly, predicts the subsequent onset of overt HE.[11] Such has been the impact of these

Division of Gastroenterology, MetroHealth Medical Center, Case Western Reserve University, 2500 MetroHealth Drive, Cleveland, OH 44109, USA
* Corresponding author.
E-mail address: kevin.mullen@case.edu

Clin Liver Dis 16 (2012) 1–5
doi:10.1016/j.cld.2012.01.001
1089-3261/12/$ – see front matter © 2012 Published by Elsevier Inc.

liver.theclinics.com

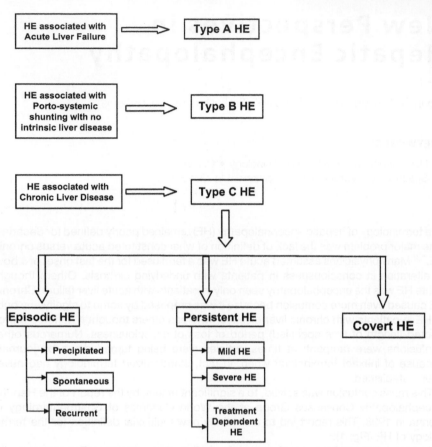

Fig. 1. Multiaxial classification of HE. This classification system was introduced by the Hepatic Encephalopathy Consensus Group at the World Congress of Gastroenterology meet in Vienna (1998). The term minimal HE is now replaced by covert HE as shown here.

findings that consideration is being given to treat patients with minimal HE before overt HE has ever occurred. Before that can be endorsed, some other issues need to be considered.

The spectrum of neurocognitive impairment in cirrhosis (SONIC) is a term coined by Bajaj and colleagues[12] to describe the prevailing status of brain function in patients with cirrhosis (Fig. 2). As noted, this concept views the spectrum as a continuum rather than as discrete, separate entities. There is good evidence for the evolution from normal mental status through minimal HE to overt HE and even potentially to hepatocerebral degeneration. Recently the term covert HE has been introduced, which encompasses the area formerly designated as minimal HE and is usually diagnosed by a psychometric test battery. However, because of the difficulty in getting standardization of what is stage I HE of New Haven scale, the authors have chosen to include this stage within the term covert HE.[13] The hepatic encephalopathy scoring algorithm and low-grade/high-grade HE distinctions have also attempted to address the problem of the subjective scoring of stage I HE on the old New Haven scale.[14,15]

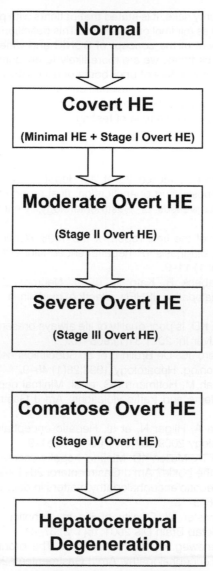

Fig. 2. Spectrum of neurocognitive impairments in cirrhosis. The range of cognitive impairments that are encountered with patients with cirrhosis from normal at one end to covert, overt, and severe irreversible stages, such as hepatocerebral degeneration, at the other. This spectrum is a continuum, and patients can fluctuate between various stages of HE based on several factors. However, development of hepatocerebral degeneration is usually irreversible.

The authors briefly mentioned the hepatocerebral syndromes (as shown in **Fig. 2**) that represent an extreme form of HE.[16] Essentially evidence of brain atrophy and microcavitation in some patients is very pronounced. Despite the damage to brain tissue, this neurodegenerative disorder does seem to be reversible, to a degree.[17] One spectacular case of brain regeneration is published in the literature, but generally far less prominent restoration of brain anatomy is noted.[18]

Conventionally, for purity sake, it is stated that patients with prior bouts of overt HE should not be classified as minimal or covert HE. This definition is only an operational definition. With the advent of the concept of SONIC and widespread psychometric testing of patients with cirrhosis, we are more likely to encounter patients who have covert HE with or without a history of prior bouts of overt HE. There is some concern that patients with prior overt HE have persistent cognitive impairments.[19] However, for all practical purposes, they should be labeled as overt, covert, or normal depending on their cognitive performance at the time of testing.

REFERENCES

1. Ferenci P, Lockwood A, Mullen K, et al. Hepatic encephalopathy–definition, nomenclature, diagnosis, and quantification: final report of the working party at the 11th World Congresses of Gastroenterology, Vienna, 1998. Hepatology 2002;35(3):716–21.
2. Mullen KD. Review of the final report of the 1998 Working Party on definition, nomenclature and diagnosis of hepatic encephalopathy. Aliment Pharmacol Ther 2007;25(Suppl 1):11–6.
3. Randolph C, Hilsabeck R, Kato A, et al. Neuropsychological assessment of hepatic encephalopathy: ISHEN practice guidelines. Liver Int 2009;29(5): 629–35.
4. Prakash RK, Mullen KD. Is poor quality of life always present with minimal hepatic encephalopathy? Liver Int 2011;31(7):908–10.
5. Groeneweg M, Quero JC, De Bruijn I, et al. Subclinical hepatic encephalopathy impairs daily functioning. Hepatology 1998;28(1):45–9.
6. Bajaj JS, Hafeezullah M, Hoffmann RG, et al. Minimal hepatic encephalopathy: a vehicle for accidents and traffic violations. Am J Gastroenterol 2007;102(9): 1903–9.
7. Kircheis G, Knoche A, Hilger N, et al. Hepatic encephalopathy and fitness to drive. Gastroenterology 2009;137(5):1706–1715.e1–9.
8. Prakash RK, Brown TA, Mullen KD. Minimal hepatic encephalopathy and driving: is the genie out of the bottle? Am J Gastroenterol 2011;106(8):1415–6.
9. Bajaj JS. Minimal hepatic encephalopathy matters in daily life. World J Gastroenterol 2008;14(23):3609–15.
10. Schomerus H, Hamster W. Quality of life in cirrhotics with minimal hepatic encephalopathy. Metab Brain Dis 2001;16(1–2):37–41.
11. Hartmann IJ, Groeneweg M, Quero JC, et al. The prognostic significance of subclinical hepatic encephalopathy. Am J Gastroenterol 2000;95(8):2029–34.
12. Bajaj JS, Wade JB, Sanyal AJ. Spectrum of neurocognitive impairment in cirrhosis: implications for the assessment of hepatic encephalopathy. Hepatology 2009;50(6):2014–21.
13. Bajaj JS, Cordoba J, Mullen KD, et al. Review article: the design of clinical trials in hepatic encephalopathy–an International Society for Hepatic Encephalopathy and Nitrogen Metabolism (ISHEN) consensus statement. Aliment Pharmacol Ther 2011;33(7):739–47.
14. Hassanein TI, Hilsabeck RC, Perry W. Introduction to the hepatic encephalopathy scoring algorithm (HESA). Dig Dis Sci 2008;53(2):529–38.
15. Haussinger D, Cordoba Cardona J, Kircheis G, et al. Definition and assessment of low-grade hepatic encephalopathy. In: Haussinger D, Kircheis G, Schliess F, editors. Hepatic encephalopathy and nitrogen metabolism. Dordrecht (Netherlands): Springer-Verlag; 2006. p. 423–32.

16. Adams RD, Foley JM. The neurological disorder associated with liver disease. Res Publ Assoc Res Nerv Ment Dis 1953;32:198–237.
17. Weissenborn K, Tietge UJ, Bokemeyer M, et al. Liver transplantation improves hepatic myelopathy: evidence by three cases. Gastroenterology 2003;124(2): 346–51.
18. Stracciari A, Guarino M, Pazzagalia P, et al. Acquired hepatocerebral degeneration: full recovery after liver transplantation. J Neurol Neurosurg Psychiatry 2001; 70(1):136–7.
19. Bajaj JS, Schubert CM, Heuman DM, et al. Persistence of cognitive impairment after resolution of overt hepatic encephalopathy. Gastroenterology 2010;138(7): 2332–40.

Theories of the Pathogenesis of Hepatic Encephalopathy

E. Anthony Jones, MD, DSc, Kevin D. Mullen, MD, FRCPI*

KEYWORDS

- Hepatic encephalopathy • Ammonia • GABA
- GABA$_A$ receptor complex

A normally functioning liver is necessary to maintain optimal brain function. The syndrome of hepatic encephalopathy (HE) or portal-systemic encephalopathy (PSE) is a complication of hepatocellular failure associated with a variable degree of shunting through portal-systemic venous collaterals.[1] Theoretically, HE may occur as a consequence of (1) reduced synthesis by the failing liver of substances necessary for normal brain function; (2) synthesis by the failing liver of encephalopathogenic substances or their precursors; and/or (3) reduced extraction and/or metabolism by the failing liver of encephalopathogenic substances or their precursors. Most research on the pathogenesis of HE has focused on the last of these possibilities.

For many centuries a relationship between the liver and mental function has been recognized.[2] However, it was not until the advent of clinical science in the mid–twentieth century that the syndrome of HE was described as a reversible metabolic encephalopathy characterized by a wide variety of neuropsychological abnormalities, including progressive impairment of consciousness, which occurred as a complication of acute or chronic hepatocellular failure.[3,4] Initially, an attempt was made to explain how increased portal-systemic shunting might contribute to the development of HE in a patient with decompensated cirrhosis. It was suggested that, in normal subjects, neuroactive substances that originate in the intestine are absorbed and subsequently metabolized by the liver. In contrast, in patients with decompensated cirrhosis, it was assumed that there would be increased delivery of such neuroactive substances to the systemic circulation as a consequence of their inadequate metabolism by the failing liver and their bypassing the liver through intrahepatic and extrahepatic portal-systemic venous collaterals. It was also assumed that increased levels of neuroactive

Division of Gastroenterology, MetroHealth Medical Center, Case Western Reserve University, 2500 MetroHealth Drive, Cleveland, OH 44109, USA
* Corresponding author.
E-mail address: kevin.mullen@case.edu

Clin Liver Dis 16 (2012) 7–26
doi:10.1016/j.cld.2011.12.010
1089-3261/12/$ – see front matter © 2012 Published by Elsevier Inc.

substances in the systemic circulation (if nonpolar and lipid soluble), would facilitate their passage across the blood-brain-barrier and access to the brain where they might induce a cerebral disturbance (**Fig. 1**).[5] In recent years, experience with transjugular intrahepatic portal-systemic shunts has reemphasized the importance of portal-systemic shunting in the pathogenesis of HE in patients with cirrhosis.[6] In general, the larger the diameter of a shunt and the greater the degree to which portal flow is less hepatopetal and more hepatofugal, then the greater the risk or severity of HE.

Increasing familiarity with the syndrome rapidly led clinicians to recognize factors that tend to precipitate HE in patients with cirrhosis (**Table 1**). Knowledge of such factors is of crucial importance in the management of patients with liver disease. However, the precise relationships between most of these factors and the mechanisms by which they contribute to HE are poorly understood. Definitive clarification of how specific factors act to precipitate HE may provide new insights into the pathogenesis of HE.

The pathophysiologic events that mediate HE occur in the brain. Originally, the neuroactive substances postulated to be involved in HE were classified as neuro-toxins, but their toxic effects on the brain were not specified. No serious attempt was made initially to define which specific neural mechanisms might be responsible for mediating the clinical features of HE,[1] and the extent to which altered brain function in HE may occur as a consequence of an increase or decrease in specific neuronal

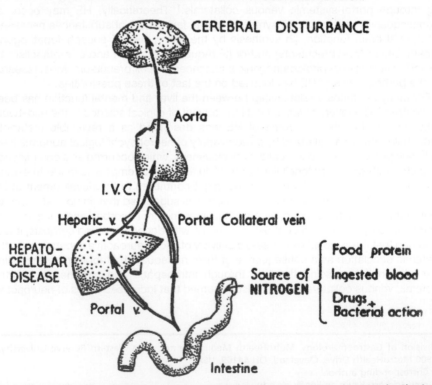

HEPATIC ENCEPHALOPATHY AND NITROGEN METABOLISM

CEREBRAL DISTURBANCE

Aorta

I.V.C.

Hepatic v.   Portal Collateral vein

HEPATO-
CELLULAR
DISEASE

Source of
NITROGEN

Food protein

Ingested blood

Drugs +
Bacterial action

Portal v.

Intestine

Fig. 1. The mechanism of portal–systemic encephalopathy, as envisioned in 1954 by Sherlock et al. See text for a description of the principal relevant concepts. (*From* Sherlock S, Summerskill WHJ, White LP, Phear EA. Portal-systemic encephalopathy: neurological complications of liver disease. Lancet 1954;264:453–7; with permission.)

Table 1 Factors that may precipitate HE	
Oral protein load Upper gastrointestinal bleed Constipation	Act through gut factors
Diarrhea and vomiting Diuretic therapy Abdominal paracentesis	Dehydration, electrolyte and acid/base imbalance (eg, hypokalemic alkalosis)
Hypoxia Hypotension Anemia Hypoglycemia	Adverse effects on both liver and brain
Sedative or hypnotic drugs[a] Azotemia[b] Infection[c] Creation of portal-systemic shunt 　General surgery	

Abbreviation: GABA$_A$, γ-aminobutyric acid type A.
[a] Includes drugs acting on the GABA$_A$/benzodiazepine receptor complex.
[b] Blood urea is a source of intestinal ammonia.
[c] May cause dehydration and increased release of nitrogenous substances.

mechanisms mediated by physiologic substances (neurotransmitters) did not receive serious consideration.

This article concentrates on classic, uncomplicated, overt HE. It does not discuss minimal or subclinical HE, the mechanisms of which may not necessarily be identical to those responsible for overt HE. In addition, in patients with cirrhosis, neurologic complications of chronic PSE, which, in contrast with classic HE, are irreversible, such as transverse myelitis and nonwilsonian hepatocerebral degeneration,[7] are not included. Complications of acute hepatocellular failure, such as increased intracranial pressure and cerebral edema,[8] are also not included, because factors not involved in the pathogenesis of HE may contribute to their development. Furthermore, aberrant findings obtained using animal models that do not meet acceptably strict criteria for defining HE are not discussed, such as the portacaval-shunted rat.[9]

THE AMMONIA HYPOTHESIS

The first and best-known theory postulates a causal relationship between increased levels of ammonia and the development of HE.[10] Ammonia is a normal physiologic product of intermediary metabolism. Major sources of plasma ammonia are the gastrointestinal tract and skeletal muscle. It is converted into urea and glutamine in the liver and into glutamine in skeletal muscle and the brain.[11,12]

In 1896, dogs with a surgically induced Eck fistula (portal-systemic shunt) were reported to exhibit neuropsychological changes that correlated with impaired detoxification of ammonia by the liver.[13] In the 1950s, an association between HE and increased blood ammonia levels was confirmed,[14,15] and the precipitation of HE in patients with cirrhosis and ascites by treatment with ammonium ion exchange resins was reported.[16] Such treatment would be expected to increase blood ammonia levels, but might also induce constipation, one of the recognized precipitating factors of HE (see **Table 1**). Early observations that were considered to support the ammonia hypothesis included not only the tendency for plasma ammonia levels to be increased in patients with chronic hepatocellular failure,[14,15] but also the recognition that ammonia mediates neurologic effects, which include convulsions,[17] and (being nonionic and lipid soluble) traverses the blood-brain barrier readily.[18] This hypothesis stimulated several elegant clinical studies of ammonia metabolism in patients with liver disease.[18–20]

However, for many years after this hypothesis was first postulated, the neural mechanisms by which ammonia might contribute to the manifestations of HE remained undefined. It seems likely that progress in characterizing such mechanisms might have been promoted by early resolution of several issues of concern. These included (1) plasma ammonia levels correlate poorly with the severity of HE[10,15]; (2) in contrast with the manifestations of increasingly severe HE, progressive acute intoxication with ammonia is characterized by a lethargic preconvulsive state, seizures, and postictal coma[21]; (3) seizures rarely occur in patients with chronic hepatocellular failure[10]; (4) in patients with chronic hepatocellular disease, EEG changes induced by administering ammonium acetate are not typical of those associated with HE[22]; (5) the neuro-electrophysiologic changes induced by ammonia in normal animals differ from those that occur in animal models of fulminant hepatic failure (FHF; ie, acute liver failure with HE)[21,23,24]; (6) hemodialysis, which reduces plasma ammonia levels, is associated with inconsistent ameliorations of HE[25]; (7) many of the neurologic effects of ammonia occur at concentrations substantially higher than those observed in humans with HE[17]; and (8) ammonia intoxication is not associated with the subtle changes in personality and mental function and inverted sleep rhythm that are characteristic features of early HE (stages 0–II) complicating chronic hepatocellular failure.[1,26]

VARIANTS OF THE AMMONIA HYPOTHESIS
Synergistic Neurotoxins

It was proposed that HE might arise as a consequence of the synergistic actions of more than 1 neurotoxin on the brain; those specified were ammonia, mercaptans, and fatty acids.[27] However, the abnormal patterns of visual evoked potentials (VEPs) that develop in a rabbit model of FHF did not resemble those induced in normal animals by administering a mixture of the synergistic neurotoxins specified.[21,23] The validity of this hypothesis is difficult to prove and convincing evidence that supports it has not materialized.

Decreased Cerebral Energy Metabolism

Evidence consistent with the occurrence of decreased cerebral energy metabolism in HE has been reported and it has been suggested that increased ammonia levels in hepatocellular failure may depress cerebral energy metabolism.[28,29] Hyperammonemia has been shown to be associated with changes in cerebral energy metabolism.[11,30] However, such changes may not contribute directly to HE and may be secondary phenomena.

OTHER HYPOTHESES

For many years after the emergence of the ammonia hypothesis, attempts to postulate causal relationships between specific hepatocellular failure–associated changes in peripheral metabolism and HE were popular; such changes included those relating to colonic metabolism of nitrogenous substances. In contrast with the ammonia hypothesis, many attempts to implicate a variety of other individual substances in the pathogenesis of HE have been proposed, but have not led to the development of any robust new theory that merits serious experimental evaluation.

THEORIES THAT IMPLICATE ALTERED NEUROTRANSMISSION

In the 1970s and the early 1980s, the main thrust of research on the pathogenesis of HE began to undergo significant changes. Increasing emphasis began to be directed toward elucidating the changes associated with hepatocellular failure that occur in neuronal mechanisms in the brain, the end organ of HE. This evolution in the approach to research on HE was associated with an increasing trend to supplement neurochemical findings with behavioral and electrophysiologic data. The new era in research on the pathogenesis of HE was summarized in an article entitled, *In hepatic coma, the problem comes from the colon, but will the answer come from there?*[31]

FALSE NEUROTRANSMITTERS AND AMINO ACID IMBALANCE

Hypotheses were proposed that implicated false neurotransmitters and the central effects of amino acid imbalance in the mediation of HE.[32–34] These hypotheses were important because they raised the possibility of a particular neural mechanism in the brain being involved in the pathogenesis of HE, specifically altered dopaminergic neurotransmission. They led to the introduction of drugs that act as agonists at dopamine receptors in the brain, in particular levadopa and bromocriptine, as well as branched-chain amino acids, as potential new therapies for HE. However, the efficacy of these proposed therapies in the management of HE was not established,[35,36] and none of them has a place in the current management of HE. Furthermore, experimental evidence that provides strong support for these hypotheses has not been forthcoming.

γ-AMINOBUTYRIC ACID–MEDIATED INHIBITORY NEUROTRANSMISSION

The γ-aminobutyric acid type A (GABA$_A$) receptor complex is the principal inhibitory neurotransmitter system of the mammalian brain (**Fig. 2**).[37] That increased GABA-mediated inhibitory neurotransmission might contribute to the manifestations of HE was first suggested by the finding that the abnormal patterns of VEPs in an animal model of FHF resembled those induced in normal animals by administration of drugs that act by enhancing GABAergic tone (GABA-mediated inhibitory neurotransmission),[23,38] such as a barbiturate or a central benzodiazepine (BZ) receptor agonist.[37] The hypothesis did not depend on any particular change in the status of receptors on the GABA$_A$ receptor complex. The functional status of this complex has been studied more extensively in models of HE than any other neurotransmitter system.[39] The hypothesis implicating this system[38] provided a potential explanation for neuropsychiatric manifestations of HE; specifically, an increase in GABA-mediated inhibitory neurotransmission is associated with decreased consciousness and impaired motor function, 2 of the classic features of the clinical syndrome of HE.[1] In contrast, a net decrease in GABA-mediated inhibitory neurotransmission is associated with increased neural excitation and the risk of seizures.[40] The GABA hypothesis raised 2 important questions. First, is there evidence that supports an increase in GABAergic tone in HE, and, second, if there is, what mechanisms could be responsible for this phenomenon?

Evidence Supporting Increased GABAergic Tone in HE

1. 3-Mercaptoproprionic acid (MPA) is an inhibitor of L-glutamate decarboxylase, which catalyzes the synthesis of GABA from glutamate. A rat model of FHF had increased resistance to the induction of seizures by the central administration of MPA.[41] Similarly, a rabbit model of FHF had increased resistance to the

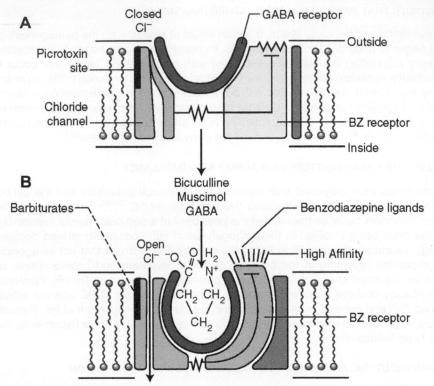

Fig. 2. The GABAA/benzodiazepine receptor-chloride ionophore complex. Receptors are depicted for GABA, barbiturates and benzodiazepine ligands. GABA receptor agonists (e.g. GABA, muscimol), and GABA receptor antagonists (e.g. bicuculline) bind to GABA g receptors; barbiturates are thought to bind to specific recognition sites near the chloride ionophore; benzodiazepine receptor agonists (e.g. diazepam), benzodiazepine receptor antagonists (e.g. flumazenil), and benzodiazepine receptor inverse agonists (e.g. 6,7 dimethoxy-4-ethyl-3-carbomethoxy-fl-carboline) bind to benzodiazepine receptors. A: shows the receptor complex in an inactivated state with the C1- channel closed. B: shows the receptor complex in an activated state with the C! channel open. Activation is induced by GABA or GABA agonists binding to GABA receptors, or by barbiturates. Activation of the receptor complex is associated with conformational changes and the opening of the Cl channel. Consequent entry of C1- into the neuron results in hyperpolarization. The frequency of chloride channel opening in the presence of GABA is increased by BZ receptor agonists. (*From* Jones AE, Basile AS, Mullen D, et al. Flumazenil: Potential Implications for Hepatic Encephalopathy. Pharmac Ther 1990;45:331–43; with permission.)

induction of seizures by the administration of the $GABA_A$ receptor antagonist, bicuculline.[42]

2. The abnormal patterns of VEPs in animal models of FHF are similar to those induced in normal animals by encephalopathogenic doses of drugs that act by augmenting GABAergic neurotransmission,[23,24,42] such as a barbiturate, a central BZ receptor agonist, or a $GABA_A$ receptor agonist.[37]

3. The spontaneous activity (discharges per second measured using a rate meter) of individual Purkinje neurons in situ in cerebellar slices from a rabbit model of FHF and control rabbits were recorded during exposure to different concentrations of the GABA agonist, muscimol. The sigmoid-shaped concentration-response curve for

Purkinje neurons from the model was shifted to the left of that for controls, indicating that, in HE, neurons exhibit increased sensitivity to depression by a GABA agonist.[43]

4. Antagonists of the GABA$_A$-BZ receptor complex, such as the GABA$_A$ receptor antagonist bicuculline, and the GABA$_A$ receptor Cl$^-$ channel blocker isopropylbicyclophosphorothionate, ameliorate behavioral and neuroelectrophysiologic deficits in a rabbit model of FHF.[42,44] In this model, in which, electrophysiologically, there was a consistent increase in the magnitude of the first negative wave of the VEP, P2, the central BZ receptor antagonist, flumazenil, not only induced behavioral ameliorations of HE but also normalized the pathologic increase in the amplitude of P2.[42]

5. In a rat model of HE, increased neuronal synthesis of GABA has been shown; such synthesis involves the indirect pathway, including the tricarboxylic acid cycle, which is stimulated by ammonia. Increased synthesis of GABA by cocultures of neurons and astrocytes exposed to ammonia was also shown.[45] These observations are consistent with HE being associated with increased GABAergic tone (discussed later).

Summary

Thus, in animal models of HE, 5 distinct observations are compatible with increased GABAergic tone: (1) increased resistance to drugs that decrease GABAergic tone; (2) abnormal VEP patterns that resemble those induced by drugs that enhance GABAergic tone; (3) increased sensitivity of central nervous system neurons to depression by a GABA agonist; (4) behavioral and electrophysiologic ameliorations of encephalopathy induced by antagonizing individual components of the GABA$_A$ receptor complex; and (5) increased neuronal synthesis of GABA.

Potential Mechanisms of Increased GABAergic Tone in HE

Increased synaptic availability of GABA

Normally, the permeability of the blood-brain barrier to nonlipid soluble polar substances, such as GABA, is low. However, the permeability of this barrier changes in acute hepatocellular failure. Using radiolabeled α-aminoisobutyric acid, a nonmetabolized polar amino acid, a substantial increase in plasma-to-brain transfer of this marker of GABA was shown in a rabbit model of FHF by quantitative autoradiography. The increased transfer was specific for brain gray matter and preceded the development of overt HE.[46] In addition, measurements of the brain uptake index of radiolabeled GABA in the same model, using the Oldendorf technique, indicated that brain uptake was higher in stage II HE than in control animals and that uptake was substantially higher in stage III than in stage II HE, with or without correction of the data for intravascular retention of labeled GABA. The methodology adopted also minimized problems attributable to the rapid metabolism of labeled GABA and slow brain washout and recirculation of the radiolabeled tracers used in the study.[47] Furthermore, decreased brain activity of GABA transaminase has been found in a rabbit model of HE,[48] and increased release of cortical GABA by cerebellar cortical slices has been shown in a rat model of HE,[49] a phenomenon that may be attributable to an associated loss of presynaptic feedback inhibition of the release of cortical GABA caused by loss of presynaptic GABA$_B$ receptors.[50] All of these findings are consistent with increased levels of synaptic GABA in liver failure.

Accumulation of natural benzodiazepines

Binding of an agonist ligand to the central BZ receptor induces conformational changes in the GABA$_A$ receptor complex that potentiate the action of GABA (see **Fig. 2**).[37]

That BZ receptor ligands with agonist properties may contribute to increased GABAergic tone in HE was originally suggested by anecdotal observations of ameliorations of clinical and electrophysiologic manifestations of HE in patients with cirrhosis or FHF induced by the intravenous administration of flumazenil (Ro 15-1788), a central BZ receptor antagonist with weak partial agonist properties.[51,52] The ability of flumazenil to induce partial transient clinical and electrophysiologic ameliorations of HE in patients with HE secondary to acute or chronic hepatocellular failure was confirmed.[53–55] This finding raised the possibility that, in HE, central BZ receptors are occupied by agonist ligands that contribute to the manifestations of HE by enhancing the action of GABA.[56,57] The effect of flumazenil in this context would be to dysinhibit neurons, thereby increasing their spontaneous activity, as a consequence of displacement of agonist ligands from central BZ receptors.

Central BZ antagonists with partial inverse agonist properties, specifically sarmazenil (Ro 15-3505) and Ro 15-4513, at doses that induce minimal behavioral and neuroelectrophysiologic effects in normal animals, have been shown to induce more complete ameliorations of HE than flumazenil in animal models of FHF.[58,59] These observations also suggest that central BZ receptor agonist ligands are present in HE. However, another mechanism that could contribute to a central BZ receptor antagonist with partial inverse agonist properties ameliorating HE is suggested by the demonstration in cultured hippocampal neurons that Ro 15-4513 inhibited increased GABA activity mediated by allopregnenolone, a neurosteroid that is a positive allosteric modulator (agonist) of the $GABA_A$ receptor[60] (discussed later).

An understanding of the characteristics of flumazenil-induced ameliorations of HE is necessary to appreciate the significance of this phenomenon in relation to the pathogenesis of HE. The short duration of flumazenil-induced ameliorations of HE is consistent with the pharmacokinetics of the drug. A lack of response of encephalopathy associated with liver disease to flumazenil can be attributed to any of several different potential explanations, such as application of inappropriate criteria to diagnose HE, use of an inappropriate animal model of HE, presence of encephalopathies other than HE, development of increased intracranial pressure and/or cerebral edema, and/or progression of liver disease to terminal hepatocellular failure.[61] In addition, a partial response of HE to flumazenil may be attributed to its weak partial agonist properties and to the likelihood that the presence in the brain of natural BZ agonist ligands is only 1 of the causes of increased GABAergic tone in HE. Failure to be aware of these potential explanations for different types of response of encephalopathy associated with liver disease to flumazenil is liable to lead to misinterpretations of results of studies of the effects of this drug on HE.

Brain extracts from a rat model of FHF were found to be 3 times more potent in inhibiting radiolabeled flumazenil binding to central BZ receptors than corresponding control extracts. GABA significantly enhanced the potency of extracts from the model in inhibiting radiolabeled flumazenil binding (positive GABA shift), indicating that these extracts contained central BZ receptor ligands with agonist properties.[62] In an autoradiographic study, binding of radiolabeled central BZ receptor ligands (flunitrazepam and flumazenil) to cerebral cortex of unwashed brain sections from a rabbit model of FHF was about 30% less than corresponding binding to unwashed control sections or washed sections from the model or control animals. Incubation with muscimol and NaCl further decreased the binding of labeled flumazenil to cortex in unwashed brain sections from the model (positive GABA shift), indicating the presence of reversible central BZ receptor ligands with agonist properties in the brain of the model.[63]

The concentrations of substances that inhibit radioligand binding to central BZ receptors were fourfold to sixfold higher in brain extracts from a rat model of FHF than in control brain extracts. High-pressure liquid chromatography (HPLC) revealed retention peaks in brain extracts from the model that corresponded with known

1,4-BZs. Mass spectroscopy confirmed the presence of diazepam and N-desmethyl-diazepam in these extracts. Mass spectroscopy and radiometric techniques indicated that the concentrations of diazepam and N-desmethyldiazepam were 5 to 7 and 2 to 9 times higher in brain extracts from the model than in control brain extracts, respectively.[64] Corresponding findings in a rabbit model of FHF were similar.[65] In patients, who died of FHF caused by acetaminophen overdose and who had not received pharmaceutical BZs, chromatographic analysis of frontal cortex revealed 4 to 19 peaks of substances that inhibited the binding of radiolabeled flumazenil to central BZ receptors, and several of the peaks had HPLC retention times that corresponded with known 1,4-BZs. Ultraviolet and mass-spectroscopic analysis confirmed that 2 of the HPLC peaks represented diazepam and N-desmethyldiazepam. A proportion of the patients had total brain BZ receptor ligand concentrations that were twofold to tenfold higher than those in control brains.[66] Thus, brain concentrations of substances that inhibit the binding of radiolabeled flumazenil to central BZ receptors are increased in some patients with FHF.

The sources of nonpharmaceutical BZs associated with HE are unknown. Intestinal bacteria seem to synthesize precursors of BZs[67] and BZs have been shown to be present in low concentrations in a variety of foods.[61] The adjective natural, rather than endogenous, has been applied to nonpharmaceutical BZs that do not seem to be synthesized in the mammalian body. The potential contribution of natural BZ receptor ligands to increased GABAergic tone in HE has recently been reviewed in detail.[61]

Studies of the effects of GABA$_A$ receptor and central BZ receptor ligands on the spontaneous firing rate of individual Purkinje neurons in situ in cerebellar slices from a rabbit model of FHF and control animals (single neuron in situ electrophysiology) have provided additional insights into the status of the GABA$_A$ receptor complex in HE. In these experiments, the calcium and magnesium ion contents of the medium were adjusted to inhibit evoked synaptic activity. Not only do neurons from the model of HE exhibit increased sensitivity to depression of their spontaneous activity by muscimol, they also exhibit increased sensitivity to depression of their spontaneous activity by a central BZ receptor agonist (flunitrazepam).[43] This phenomenon at the cellular level seems to be analogous to the finding that patients with cirrhosis and impaired hepatocellular function exhibit hypersensitivity of the brain to the neuroinhibitory effects of a central BZ receptor agonist (triazolam).[68] When Purkinje neurons from the model of HE were exposed to central BZ receptor antagonists (flumazenil or Ro 14-7437) there were striking concentration-dependent increases in their spontaneous firing rate, whereas the same drugs did not increase the firing rate of control neurons.[43] Flumazenil induced a concentration-dependent decrease in the spontaneous firing rate of control neurons, because of its partial agonist properties.[43] The increased spontaneous firing rate of neurons from the model of HE induced by central BZ receptor antagonists probably represents dysinhibition of neurons caused by displacement of agonist ligands from central BZ receptors. The increased sensitivity of Purkinje neurons from the model of HE to depression of their spontaneous activity by muscimol could be abolished by coexposure to a BZ receptor antagonist.[43] These findings suggest that hepatocellular failure is associated with the presence of a substance that increases the sensitivity of the GABA$_A$ receptor complex to agonist ligands and with an altered functional status of components of the GABA$_A$ receptor complex.

Summary

Two potential mechanisms of increased GABAergic tone in models of HE are discussed in this article: (1) increased synaptic availability of GABA, and (2) accumulation in the brain of central BZ receptor ligands with agonist properties. Potential mechanisms by which ammonia may contribute to increased GABAergic tone in HE also seem to be important and are discussed later.

Glutamate-mediated Excitatory Neurotransmission

Glutamate is the principal excitatory neurotransmitter of the mammalian brain. It has been studied in models of HE more extensively than other excitatory neurotransmitters.[69,70]

In liver failure, increased concentrations of ammonia in the brain promote the synthesis of glutamine from glutamate, a reaction catalyzed by the astrocyte-specific enzyme, glutamine synthetase.[69,70] Ammonia decreases glutamate uptake by astrocytes[71,72] and, in models of HE, there seems to be increased cortical release of glutamate,[73] and decreased astrocytic and neuronal reuptake of glutamate.[72,74] These phenomena result in increased levels of free glutamate in brain extracellular fluid.[75–78] Decreased astrocytic reuptake of glutamate is associated with decreased expression of the astroglia-specific glutamate transporter, GLT-1.[72,79] An increase in synaptic glutamate levels is expected to lead to a compensatory decrease in glutamate receptors (N-methyl-D-aspartate [NMDA], KA/AMPA) and G protein-linked metabotropic receptors. In some models of HE, glutamate receptors have been reported to be reduced in certain brain regions.[80–84] A decreased density of glutamate receptors in liver failure may be associated with decreased glutamate-mediated excitatory neurotransmission, a phenomenon that might contribute to a net increase in inhibitory neurotransmission, and, consequently, to the manifestations of HE. In addition, ammonia (1 mM) decreases the electrophysiologic responsiveness of postsynaptic glutamate receptors,[85–87] a phenomenon that may also contribute to decreased excitatory neurotransmission.

In a rat model of FHF, administration of the competitive antagonist of a subclass of glutamate receptors (NMDA), memantine, was associated with behavioral and electrophysiologic ameliorations of encephalopathy and reduced accumulation of glutamate in cerebrospinal fluid.[88] The appropriateness of the model used and the implications of these findings for human FHF are uncertain.

The occurrence of seizures during the course of FHF may result from a rapid increase in ammonia to levels that induce neuronal excitation,[17] or from increased glutamatergic excitatory neurotransmission caused by increased synaptic concentrations of glutamate.

Imbalance Between Inhibitory and Excitatory Neurotransmission

Because the effects of a decrease in glutamatergic tone are similar to those of an increase in inhibitory neurotransmission, manifestations of HE could arise as a consequence of an imbalance between the activities of inhibitory and excitatory neurotransmitter systems that result in a net increase in inhibitory neurotransmission. In this context some manifestations of HE may be explained by disturbances in the functional loops of basal ganglia, which could arise from an imbalance between glutamatergic and GABAergic neurotransmission.[1]

Other Neurotransmitters

Roles for other neurotransmitter systems in HE have been suggested, but not yet confirmed.[89–96]

THE AMMONIA HYPOTHESIS REVISITED

As research on the pathogenesis of HE has focused increasingly on the potential relevance of altered neural mechanisms in the brain,[31] it has become relevant to assess whether the effects of ammonia on the brain include changes in the functional status of specific neural mechanisms that could potentially contribute to the manifestations of HE. In this context, the prevailing concentration of ammonia seems to be critical. An evaluation of issues of concern with the ammonia hypothesis, such as those mentioned on the ammonia hypothesis, should include an appraisal of the particular ranges of ammonia concentrations that are associated with specific phenomena, paying special attention to phenomena associated with the mildly increased ammonia concentrations, within the pathophysiologic range, that occur in patients with hepatocellular failure.[97]

Significance of Ammonia Concentrations

Plasma ammonia concentrations higher than those usually found in patients with chronic hepatocellular failure are associated with effects that do not mimic HE. In particular, concentrations of 0.75 to 1.5 mM have been shown to activate chloride extrusion pumps, suppress inhibitory postsynaptic potential formation, and depolarize neurons[98]; these effects are neuroexcitatory and their behavioral manifestations, which include seizures, do not resemble HE.[39,97,99] These phenomena occur at ammonia concentrations found in patients with congenital hyperammonemias,[26,97] and adequately explain the clinical features of these syndromes. The question arises whether the modestly increased plasma ammonia concentrations (0.1–0.75 mM) typically found in patients with precoma HE (stages I–III)[97] enhance inhibitory neurotransmission and contribute to the cognitive and motor deficits of HE.

Direct Effect of Ammonia on the GABA_A Receptor

The relative change of GABA-induced Cl^- current in cultured dispersed rat cortical neurons was studied in the presence of different concentrations of ammonia. Ionic currents were recorded using a patch clamp amplifier and were monitored simultaneously on a storage oscilloscope and a thermal-head pen recorder. Ammonia alone had little effect on the current. However, in the presence of GABA (10^{-5} M), ammonia at concentrations of 0.1 to 0.5 mM, which have minimal effects on neuronal resting potential or polarization,[98] induced a concentration-dependent increase in GABA-induced Cl^- current, as a consequence of a direct interaction between ammonia and a binding site for ammonia on the GABA_A receptor complex (**Fig. 3**).[100] This effect occurred at ammonia concentrations that commonly occur in patients with precoma HE (stages I–III),[97] and may be attributable to ammonia increasing the affinity of the GABA_A receptor to GABA.[100] This phenomenon was not modulated by flumazenil, suggesting that it was not mediated by the central BZ receptor.[100] Higher concentrations of ammonia (>1.0 mM) did not increase GABA-induced Cl^- current further.[100] Thus, the ammonia concentrations that occur in liver failure may directly enhance the ability of GABA to depress neuronal activity by modifying the affinity of the GABA_A receptor for GABA. The mechanisms underlying the direct actions of ammonia on the GABA_A receptor complex resemble those underlying the actions of barbiturates.[101]

Synergistic Interaction Between Ammonia and Agonist Ligands of the GABA_A Receptor Complex

Using radioligand binding assays, the effects of ammonia on the binding of ligands to the GABA_A receptor complex were shown to be biphasic. Ammonia, at concentrations of 0.05 to 0.5 mM, induced a concentration-dependent increase in the maximal binding of muscimol to the GABA_A receptor. Further increases in ammonia concentrations, from 0.75 to 2 mM, returned muscimol binding to control levels. Binding of a GABA_A receptor antagonist was not affected by ammonia (**Fig. 4**).[102] Ammonia at concentrations of 0.05 to 0.5 mM also induced a concentration-dependent increase

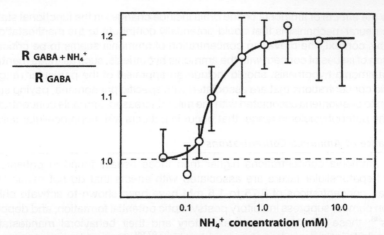

Fig. 3. Concentration–response relationship for the enhancement of 10–5 M GABA-induced chloride current by ammonium ion in dissociated rat cortical neurons. The vertical axis is the potentiation ratio. Each point is the mean of 5–9 experiments. Vertical bars indicate ± S.E.M. Neurons were pre-treated for 60 s with ammonium ion at various concentrations. (*From* Takahashi K, Kameda H, Kataoka M, et al. Ammonia potentiates GABA$_A$ response in dissociated rat cortical neurons. Neuroscience Letters 1993;151:51–4; with permission.)

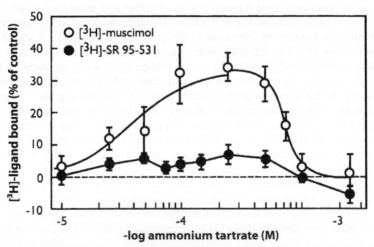

Fig. 4. Ammonium tartrate-induced modulation of radioligand binding to the GABAA receptor on rat brain membrane preparations. Data on the binding of the GABA agonist, muscimol, and the GABA antagonist, SR 05-531, are shown. Ammonium tartrate (10–500 M) significantly (33%) increased the Emax of 500nM [3H]-muscimol binding above control levels (EC50 40 M). Increasing the ammonium tartrate concentration further (500 M to 2.5 mM) lowered the binding of 500 nM [3H]-muscimol to control levels. In contrast, ammonium tartrate did not significantly modify the binding of 500 nM [3H]-SR 95-531. (*From* Ha J-H, Basile AS. Modulation of ligand binding to components of the GABA$_A$ receptor complex by ammonia: implications for the pathogenesis of hyperammonemic syndromes. Brain Research 1996;720:35–44; with permission.)

in binding of the central BZ receptor agonist, flunitrazepam, to central BZ receptors, but further increases in ammonia concentrations (0.75–2 mM) returned flunitrazepam binding to control levels. GABA itself was shown to enhance ammonia-induced increases in the binding of flumazenil to central BZ receptors.[102] These synergistic effects of ammonia on the binding of agonist ligands to the GABA$_A$ receptor complex are expected to enhance GABAergic tone.

Ammonia and Brain Extracellular Concentrations of GABA

Acute exposure to ammonia and exposure to ammonia for 4 days have been shown to promote GABA release and to induce concentration-dependent decreases in GABA uptake by cultured astrocytes. Inhibition of GABA uptake was associated with a marked decrease in V_{max} and a smaller decrease in the Michaelis constant (K_m).[103] The concentrations of ammonia that mediated these effects included those within the range associated with hepatocellular failure in patients. Thus, in hepatocellular failure, ammonia may contribute to increased synaptic availability of GABA.

Ammonia and Neurosteroids

Ammonia may enhance GABA-mediated neurotransmission in hepatocellular failure as a consequence of its effects on the peripheral-type BZ receptor (PTBR). The PTBR is located in the outer mitochondrial membrane of astrocytes.[104–106] These receptors are upregulated by ammonia in cultured astrocyes,[107] and they are upregulated in a model of FHF[108,109] and in brain autopsy samples from patients with cirrhosis who had HE terminally.[110] Upregulation of the astrocytic PTBR promotes transport of cholesterol across the mitochondrial membrane, astrocytic mitochondrial synthesis of neurosteroids from cholesterol, and subsequent release of neurosteroids into the brain extracellular space.[108,111–114] Neurosteroids bind to specific sites on the GABA$_A$ receptor complex that are distinct from BZ and barbiturate binding sites.[37,115–118] Neurosteroids include the most potent known agonists (positive allosteric modulators) of the GABA$_A$ receptor complex, for example, tetrahydroprogesterone (THP) and tetrahydrodeoxycorticosterone (THDOC).[115,117,118] Thus, in liver failure, increased binding of neurosteroid agonists to the GABA$_A$ receptor complex may occur as a consequence of ammonia-induced upregulation of PTBRs, leading to increased synthesis and release of neurosteroids. Increased brain levels of THP and THDOC have been found in a model of FHF, and, when THP or THDOC was injected into normal mice, sedation was induced.[108,114] Furthermore, increased levels of allopregnenolone, a positive allosteric modulator of the GABA$_A$ receptor, have been found in autopsied brain of cirrhotic patients who developed HE terminally.[119] In addition, the endogenous neurosteroid antagonist pregnenolone sulfate,[120] which antagonizes the neurosteroid binding site on the GABA$_A$ receptor complex, reduces the mortality associated with hyperammonemia or acute hepatocellular failure in mice.[121] These findings raise the possibility that, in liver failure, increased concentrations of ammonia may increase PTBR-mediated astrocytic synthesis and release of potent neurosteroid enhancers of GABAergic neurotransmission, and hence contribute to HE.[70,97,122–126]

SUMMARY

Ammonia and GABAergic neurotransmission seem to be interrelated factors in the pathogenesis of HE.

REFERENCES

1. Jones EA, Weissenborn K. Neurology and the liver. In: Hughes RA, Perkin GD, editors. Neurology and medicine. London: BMJ Books; 1999. p. 240–77.

2. Frerichs FT. Translated by Murchison C. A clinical treatise on diseases of the liver, vol. 1. London: New Sydenham Society; 1960. p. 193–246.
3. Adams RD, Foley JM. The neurological disorders associated with liver disease. Res Publ Assoc Res Nerv Ment Dis 1953;32:198–237.
4. Davidson EA, Summerskill WH. Psychiatric aspects of liver disease. Postgrad Med J 1956;32:487–94.
5. Sherlock S, Summerskill WH, White LP, et al. Portal-systemic encephalopathy: neurological complications of liver disease. Lancet 1954;264:453–7.
6. Nolte W, Wiltfang J, Schindler C, et al. Portosystemic hepatic encephalopathy after transjugular intrahepatic portosystemic shunt in patients with cirrhosis: clinical, laboratory, psychometric, and electroencephalographic investigations. Hepatology 1998;28:1212–25.
7. Read AE, Sherlock S, Laidlaw J, et al. The neuro-psychiatric syndromes associated with chronic liver disease and an extensive portal-systemic collateral circulation. Q J Med 1967;36:135–50.
8. Jones EA, Lavini C. Is cerebral edema a component of the syndrome of hepatic encephalopathy? Hepatology 2002;35:1270–3.
9. Mullen KD, Roessle M, Jones DB, et al. Precipitation of overt encephalopathy in the portacaval shunted rat: towards the development of an adequate model of chronic portal-systemic encephalopathy. Eur J Gastroenterol Hepatol 1997;9:293–8.
10. Conn HO, Lieberthal MM. The hepatic coma syndromes and lactulose. Baltimore (MD): Williams & Wilkins; 1978.
11. Cooper AJ, Plum F. Biochemistry and physiology of brain ammonia. Physiol Rev 1987;67:440–519.
12. Huizenga JR, Gips CH, Tangerman A. The contribution of various organs to ammonia formation: a review of factors determining the arterial ammonia concentration. Ann Clin Biochem 1996;33:23–30.
13. Nencki M, Pavlov J, Zaleski J. Uber den Ammoniakgehalt des Blutes und der Organe und die Harnstoffbildung bei den Saugetieren. Arch Exp Pathol Pharmacol 1896;37:26–51 [in German].
14. Havens LL, Child CG III. Recurrent psychosis associated with liver disease and elevated blood ammonia. N Engl J Med 1955;252:756–9.
15. Phear EA, Sherlock S, Summerskill WH. Blood ammonia levels in liver disease and 'hepatic coma'. Lancet 1955;1:836–40.
16. Gabuzda GT, Phillips GB, Davidson CS. Reversible toxic manifestations in patients with cirrhosis of the liver given cation exchange resins. N Engl J Med 1952;246:124–30.
17. Iles JF, Jack JJ. Ammonia: assessment of its action on postsynaptic inhibition as a cause of convulsions. Brain 1980;103:555–78.
18. Lockwood AH, McDonald JM, Reiman RE, et al. The dynamics of ammonia metabolism in man. Effects of liver disease and hyperammonemia. J Clin Invest 1979;63:449–60.
19. Bessman SP, Bessnam AN. The cerebral and peripheral uptake of ammonia in liver disease with an hypothesis for the mechanism of hepatic coma. J Clin Invest 1955;34:622–8.
20. Schenker S, McCandless DW, Brophy E, et al. Studies on the intracerebral toxicity of ammonia. J Clin Invest 1967;46:838–48.
21. Pappas SC, Ferenci P, Schafer DF, et al. Visual evoked potentials in a rabbit model of hepatic encephalopathy. II. Comparisons of hyperammonemic encephalopathy, postictal coma, and coma induced by synergistic neurotoxins. Gastroenterology 1984;86:546–51.

22. Cohn R, Castell DO. The effect of acute hyperammonemia on the electroencephalogram. J Lab Clin Med 1966;68:195–205.
23. Schafer DF, Pappas SC, Brody LE, et al. Visual evoked potentials in a rabbit model of hepatic encephalopathy. I. Sequential changes and comparisons with drug-induced comas. Gastroenterology 1984;86:540–5.
24. Jones DB, Mullen KD, Roessle M, et al. Hepatic encephalopathy: application of visual evoked responses to test hypotheses of its pathogenesis in rats. J Hepatol 1987;4:118–26.
25. Opolon P. Large-pore hemodialysis in fulminant hepatic failure. In: Brunner G, Schmidt FW, editors. Artificial liver support. Berlin: Springer Verlag; 1980. p. 141–6.
26. Flannery DB, Hsai E, Wolf B. Current status of hyperammonemia syndromes. Hepatology 1982;2:495–506.
27. Zieve L, Doizaki WM, Zieve FJ. Synergism between mercaptans and ammonia or fatty acids in the production of coma: a possible role for mercaptans in the pathogenesis of hepatic coma. J Lab Clin Med 1974;83:16–28.
28. Fazekas JF, Ticktin HE, Ehrmantraut WR, et al. Cerebral metabolism in hepatic insufficiency. Am J Med 1956;21:843–9.
29. McCandless DW, Schenker S. Effect of acute ammonia intoxication on energy stores in the cerebral reticular activating system. Exp Brain Res 1981;44:325–30.
30. Hawkins RA, Mans AM. Brain energy metabolism in hepatic encephalopathy. In: Butterworth RF, Pomier-Layrargues G, editors. Hepatic encephalopathy. Pathophysiology and treatment. Clifton (NJ): Humana Press; 1989. p. 159–76.
31. Schafer DF. In hepatic coma, the problem comes from the colon, but will the answer come from there? J Lab Clin Med 1987;110:253–4.
32. Fischer JE, Baldessarini RJ. False neurotransmitters and hepatic failure. Lancet 1971;2:75–80.
33. Soeters PB, Fischer JE. Insulin, glucagon, amino acid imbalance, and hepatic encephalopathy. Lancet 1976;308:880–2.
34. James JH, Ziparo V, Jeppsson B, et al. Hyperammonemia, plasma amino acid imbalance, and blood-brain amino acid transport: a unified theory of portal-systemic encephalopathy. Lancet 1979;314:772–5.
35. Als-Nielsen B, Koretz RL, Kjaergard LL, et al. Branched-chain amino acids for hepatic encephalopathy. Cochrane Database Syst Rev 2003;2:CD001939.
36. Als-Nielsen B, Gluud LL, Gluud C. Dopaminergic agents for hepatic encephalopathy. Cochrane Database Syst Rev 2004;4:CD003047.
37. MacDonald RL, Olsen RW. GABA$_A$ receptor channels. Annu Rev Neurosci 1994; 17:569–602.
38. Schafer DF, Jones EA. Hepatic encephalopathy and the gamma-aminobutyric acid neurotransmitter system. Lancet 1982;1:18–20.
39. Basile AS, Jones EA, Skolnick P. The pathogenesis and treatment of hepatic encephalopathy: evidence for the involvement of benzodiazepine receptor ligands. Pharmacol Rev 1990;43:27–71.
40. Jones EA. Benzodiazepine receptor ligands and hepatic encephalopathy: further unfolding of the GABA story. Hepatology 1991;14:1286–90.
41. Ferreira MD, Gammal SH, Jones EA. Resistance to 3-mercaptoproprionic acid-induced seizures in hepatic encephalopathy. Hepatogastroenterology 1997;44: 766–9.
42. Bassett ML, Mullen KD, Slolnick P, et al. Amelioration of hepatic encephalopathy by pharmacological antagonism of the GABA$_A$-benzodiazepine receptor complex in a rabbit model of fulminant hepatic failure. Gastroenterology 1987; 93:1069–77.

43. Basile AS, Gammal SH, Mullen KD, et al. Differential responsiveness of cerebellar Purkinje neurons to GABA and benzodiazepine receptor ligands in an animal model of hepatic encephalopathy. J Neurosci 1988;8:2414–21.
44. Gammal SH, Basile AS, Geller D, et al. Reversal of the behavioural and electrophysiological abnormalities of an animal model of hepatic encephalopathy by benzodiazepine receptor ligands. Hepatology 1990;11:371–8.
45. Leke R, Bak LK, Iversen P, et al. Synthesis of neurotransmitter GABA via the neuronal tricarboxylic acid cycle is elevated in rats with liver cirrhosis consistent with high GABAergic tone in chronic hepatic encephalopathy. J Neurochem 2011;117:824–32.
46. Horowitz ME, Schafer DF, Molnar P, et al. Increased blood-brain transfer in a rabbit model of acute liver failure. Gastroenterology 1983;84:1003–11.
47. Bassett ML, Mullen KD, Scholz B, et al. Increased brain uptake of gamma-aminobutyric acid in a rabbit model of hepatic encephalopathy. Gastroenterology 1990;98:747–57.
48. Ferenci P, Jacobs R, Pappas SC, et al. Enzymes of cerebral GABA metabolism and synaptosomal GABA uptake in acute liver failure in the rabbit. Evidence for decreased GABA-transaminase activity. J Neurochem 1984;42:1487–90.
49. Wysmuk U, Oja SS, Saransaari P, et al. Enhanced GABA release in cerebral cortical slices derived from rats with thioacetamide-induced hepatic encephalopathy. Neurochem Res 1992;17:1187–90.
50. Oja SS, Saransaari P, Wysmuk U, et al. Loss of $GABA_B$ binding sites in the cerebral cortex of rats with acute hepatic encephalopathy. Brain Res 1993;629:355–7.
51. Bansky G, Meier PJ, Ziegler WH, et al. Reversal of hepatic coma by benzodiazepine antagonist (Ro 15-1788). Lancet 1985;1:1324–5.
52. Scollo-Lavizzari G, Steinmann E. Reversal of hepatic coma by benzodiazepine antagonist (Ro 15-1788). Lancet 1985;1:1324.
53. Grimm G, Ferenci P, Katzenschlager R, et al. Improvement of hepatic encephalopathy treated with flumazenil. Lancet 1988;2:1392–4.
54. Bansky G, Meier PJ, Riederer E, et al. Effects of benzodiazepine receptor antagonist flumazenil in hepatic encephalopathy in humans. Gastroenterology 1989;97:744–50.
55. Als-Nielsen B, Gluud LL, Gluud C. Benzodiazepine receptor antagonists for hepatic encephalopathy. Cochrane Database Syst Rev 2004;2:CD002798.
56. Mullen KD, Martin JV, Mendelson WB, et al. Could an endogenous benzodiazepine ligand contribute to hepatic encephalopathy? Lancet 1988;1:457–9.
57. Jones EA, Basile AS, Mullen KD, et al. Flumazenil: potential implications for hepatic encephalopathy. Pharmacol Ther 1990;45:331–43.
58. Bosman DK, van den Buijs CA, de Haan JG, et al. The effects of benzodiazepine-receptor antagonists and partial inverse agonists on acute hepatic encephalopathy in the rat. Gastroenterology 1991;101:772–81.
59. Stendl P, Puspok A, Druml W, et al. Beneficial effect of pharmacological modulation of the $GABA_A$-benzodiazepine receptor in hepatic encephalopathy in the rat: comparison with uremic encephalopathy. Hepatology 1991;14:963–8.
60. Ahboucha S, Coyne L, Hirakawa R, et al. An interaction between benzodiazepines and neuroactive steroids at $GABA_A$ receptors in cultured hippocampal neurons. Neurochem Int 2006;48:703–7.
61. Jones EA, Mullen KD. The role of natural benzodiazepine receptor ligands in hepatic encephalopathy. In: Mullen KD, Prakash R, editors. Hepatic encephalopathy. Springer Publications, in press.

62. Basile AS, Gammal SH, Jones EA, et al. The GABA$_A$ receptor complex in an experimental model of hepatic encephalopathy: evidence for elevated levels of an endogenous benzodiazepine receptor ligand. J Neurochem 1989;53: 1057–63.

63. Basile AS, Ostrowski NL, Gammal SH, et al. The GABA$_A$ receptor complex in hepatic encephalopathy. Autoradiographic evidence for the presence of elevated levels of a benzodiazepine receptor ligand. Neuropsychopharmacology 1990;3:61–7.

64. Basile AS, Pannel L, Jaouni T, et al. Brain concentrations of benzodiazepines are elevated in an animal model of hepatic encephalopathy. Proc Natl Acad Sci U S A 1990;87:5263–7.

65. Basile AS. The contribution of endogenous benzodiazepine receptor ligands to the pathogenesis of hepatic encephalopathy. Synapse 1991;7:141–50.

66. Basile AS, Hughes RD, Harrison PM, et al. Elevated brain concentrations of 1,4-benzodiazepines in fulminant hepatic failure. N Engl J Med 1991;325:473–8.

67. Yurdaydin C, Walsh TJ, Engler HD, et al. Gut bacteria provide precursors of benzodiazepine receptor ligands in a rat model of hepatic encephalopathy. Brain Res 1995;679:42–8.

68. Bakti G, Fisch HU, Karlaganis G, et al. Mechanism of the selective response of cirrhotics to benzodiazepines. Model experiments with triazolam. Hepatology 1987;7:629–38.

69. Butterworth RF. The neurobiology of hepatic encephalopathy. Semin Liver Dis 1996;16:235–44.

70. Norenberg MD. Astrocytic-ammonia interactions in hepatic encephalopathy. Semin Liver Dis 1996;16:245–53.

71. Bender AS, Norenberg MD. Effects of ammonia on L-glutamate uptake in cultured astrocytes. Neurochem Res 1996;21:567–73.

72. Norenberg MD, Huo Z, Neary JT, et al. The glial glutamate transporter in hyper-ammonemia and hepatic encephalopathy: relation to energy metabolism and glutamatergic neurotransmission. Glia 1997;21:124–33.

73. Moroni F, Lombardi G, Moneti G, et al. The release and neosynthesis of glutamic acid are increased in experimental models of hepatic encephalopathy. J Neurochem 1983;40:850–4.

74. Oppong KN, Bartlett K, Record CO, et al. Synaptosomal glutamate transport in thioacetamide-induced hepatic encephalopathy in the rat. Hepatology 1995;22: 553–8.

75. Bosman DK, Chamuleau RA, Bovee WM, et al. The glutamate hypothesis studied by brain dialysis and ^{1}H-NMR spectroscopy in cerebral cortex of the rat during acute hepatic encephalopathy. In: Bengtsson F, Jeppson B, Almdal T, et al, editors. Progress in hepatic encephalopathy and metabolic nitrogen exchange. Boca Raton (FL): CRC Press; 1991. p. 197–209.

76. De Knegt RJ, Schalm SW, van der Rigt CC, et al. Extracellular brain glutamate during acute liver failure and during acute hyperammonemia simulating acute liver failure: an experimental study based on in vivo brain dialysis. J Hepatol 1994;20:19–26.

77. Michalak A, Rose C, Butterworth J, et al. Neuroactive amino acids and glutamate (NMDA) receptors in frontal cortex of rats with experimental acute liver failure. Hepatology 1996;24:908–13.

78. Hilgier WM, Zielinska HD, Borkowska R, et al. Changes in the extracellular profiles of neuroactive amino acids in the rat striatum at the asymptomatic stage of hepatic failure. J Neurosci Res 1999;56:76–84.

79. Knecht K, Michalak A, Rose C, et al. Decreased glutamate transporter (GLT-1) expression in frontal cortex of rats with acute liver failure. Neurosci Lett 1997; 229:201–3.
80. Ferenci P, Pappas SC, Munson PJ, et al. Changes in glutamate receptors on synaptic membranes associated with hepatic encephalopathy or hyperammonemia in the rabbit. Hepatology 1984;4:25–9.
81. Maddison JE, Watson WE, Dodd PR, et al. Alterations in cortical [^{3}H]kainite and alpha-[^{3}H]amino-3-hydroxy-5-methyl-4-isoxazolepropionic acid binding in a spontaneous canine model of chronic hepatic encephalopathy. J Neurochem 1991;56:1881–8.
82. Maddison JE, Warson WE, Johnson GA. CNQX binding to non-NMDA glutamate receptors in canine cerebro-cortical crude synaptosomal membranes: pharmacological characterization and comparison of binding parameters in dogs with congenital portosystemic encephalopathy and control dogs. Metab Brain Dis 1992;7:35–44.
83. Michalak A, Butterworth RF. Selective loss of binding sites for the glutamate receptor ligands [^{3}H]kainite and (S)-[^{3}H]5-fluorowillardine in the brains of rats with acute liver failure. Hepatology 1997;25:631–5.
84. Saransaari P, Oja SS, Borkowska HD, et al. Effects of thioacetamide-induced hepatic failure on the N-methyl-D-aspartate receptor complex in the rat cerebral cortex, striatum and hippocampus: binding of different ligands and expression of receptor subunit mRNAs. Mol Chem Neuropathol 1997;32:179–93.
85. Fan P, Lavoie J, Le NL, et al. Neurochemical and electrophysiological studies on the inhibitory effect of ammonium ions on synaptic transmission in slices of rat hippocampus: evidence for a postsynaptic action. Neuroscience 1990;37:327–34.
86. Lombardi G, Mannaioni G, Leonardi P, et al. Ammonium acetate inhibits ionotropic receptors and differentially affects metabotropic receptors for glutamate. J Neural Transm 1994;97:187–96.
87. Marcaida G, Minana MD, Burgal M, et al. Ammonia prevents activation of NMDA receptors by glutamate in rat cerebellar neuronal cultures. Eur J Neurosci 1995; 7:2389–96.
88. Vogels BA, Maas MA, Daalhuisen J, et al. Memantine, a noncompetitive NMDA receptor antagonist, improves hyperammonemia-induced encephalopathy and acute hepatic encephalopathy in rats. Hepatology 1997;25:820–7.
89. Yurdaydin C, Herneth AM, Puspok A, et al. Modulation of hepatic encephalopathy in rats with thioacetamide-induced acute liver failure by serotonin antagonists. Eur J Gastroenterol Hepatol 1996;8:667–71.
90. Mousseau DD, Baker GB, Butterworth RF. Increased density of catalytic sites and expression of brain monamine oxidase A in humans with hepatic encephalopathy. J Neurochem 1997;68:1200–8.
91. Michalak A, Rose C, Butterworth RF. Loss of noradrenaline transporter sites in frontal cortex of rats with acute (ischemic) liver failure. Neurochem Int 2001; 38:25–30.
92. Michalak A, Chatauret N, Butterworth RF. Evidence for a serotonin transporter deficit in experimental acute liver failure. Neurochem Int 2001;38:163–8.
93. Waskiewics J, Fresko I, Lenkiewicz A, et al. Reversible decrease of dopamine D2 receptor density in the striatum of rats with acute hepatic failure. Brain Res 2001;900:143–5.
94. Lozeva V, Tuomisto L, Sola D, et al. Increased density of brain histamine H(1) receptors in rats with portacaval anastomosis and in cirrhotic patients with chronic hepatic encephalopathy. Hepatology 2001;33:1370–6.

95. Lozeva V, Tuomisto L, Tarhanen J, et al. Increased concentrations of histamine and its metabolite, telemethylhistamine and down-regulation of histamine H3 receptor sites in autopsied brain tissue from cirrhotic patients who died in hepatic coma. J Hepatol 2003;39:522–7.
96. Bergasa NV, Rothman RB, Mukerjee E, et al. Up-regulation of mu-opioid receptors in a model of hepatic encephalopathy: a potential explanation for increased sensitivity to morphine in liver failure. Life Sci 2002;70:1701–8.
97. Basile AS, Jones EA. Ammonia and GABAergic neurotransmission: interrelated factors in the pathogenesis of hepatic encephalopathy. Hepatology 1997;25: 1303–5.
98. Raabe W. Neurophysiology of ammonia intoxication. In: Butterworth RF, Pomier-Layrargues G, editors. Hepatic encephalopathy. Pathophysiology and treatment. Clifton (NJ): Humana Press; 1989. p. 49–77.
99. Szerb JC, Butterworth RF. Effect of ammonium ions on synaptic transmission in the mammalian central nervous system. Prog Neurobiol 1992;39:135–53.
100. Takahashi K, Kameda H, Kataoka M, et al. Ammonia potentiates $GABA_A$ response in dissociated rat cortical neurons. Neurosci Lett 1993;151:51–4.
101. Willow M, Johnson GA. Dual action of pentobarbitone on GABA binding: role of binding site integrity. J Neurochem 1981;37:1291–4.
102. Ha JH, Basile AS. Modulation of ligand binding to components of the $GABA_A$ receptor complex by ammonia: implications for the pathogenesis of hyperammonemic syndromes. Brain Res 1996;720:35–44.
103. Bender AS, Norenberg MD. Effect of ammonia on GABA uptake and release in cultured astrocytes. Neurochem Int 2000;36:389–95.
104. Basile AS, Skolnick P. Subcellular localization of "peripheral-type" binding site for benzodiazepines in rat brain. J Neurochem 1986;46:305–8.
105. Anholt RR, Pedersen PL, DeSouza EB, et al. The peripheral-type benzodiazepine receptor: localization to the mitochondrial outer membrane. J Biol Chem 1986;261:576–83.
106. Itzak Y, Baker AS, Norenberg MD. Characterization of peripheral-type benzodiazepine receptor in cultured astrocytes. Evidence for multiplicity. Glia 1993;9:211–8.
107. Itzak Y, Norenberg MD. Ammonia induced upregulation of peripheral-type benzodiazepine receptors in cultured astrocytes labelled with [^{3}H]PK 11195. Neurosci Lett 1994;177:35–8.
108. Itzak Y, Roig-Cantisano A, Dombro RS, et al. Acute liver failure and hyperammonemia increase peripheral-type benzodiazepine receptor binding and pregnenolone synthesis in mouse brain. Brain Res 1995;705:345–8.
109. Kadota Y, Inoue K, Tokunaga R, et al. Induction of peripheral-type benzodiazepine receptors in mouse brain following thioacetamide-induced acute liver failure. Life Sci 1996;58:953–9.
110. Lavoie J, Pomier-Layrargues G, Butterworth RF. Increased densities of peripheral-type benzodiazepine receptors in brain autopsy samples from cirrhotic patients with hepatic encephalopathy. Hepatology 1990;11:874–8.
111. Krueger KE, Papadopoulos V. Mitochondrial benzodiazepine receptors and the regulation of steroid biosynthesis. Annu Rev Pharmacol 1992;32:211–37.
112. Akwa Y, Saranes N, Gouezou M, et al. Astrocytes and neurosteroids: metabolism of pregnenolone and dehydro-epiandrosterone. Regulation by cell density. J Cell Biol 1993;12:135–43.
113. Papadopoulos V. Peripheral-type benzodiazepine/diazepam binding inhibitor receptor: biological role in steroidogenic cell function. Endocr Rev 1993;14: 222–40.

114. Norenberg MD, Itzak Y, Bender AS. The peripheral benzodiazepine receptor and neurosteroids in hepatic encephalopathy. Adv Exp Med Biol 1997;420: 95–110.
115. Majewska MD, Harrison NL, Schwartz RD, et al. Steroid hormone metabolites are barbiturate-like modulators of the GABA receptor. Science 1986;232: 1004–7.
116. Turner DM, Ransom RW, Yang SJ, et al. Steroid anesthetics and naturally occurring analogs modulate the gamma-aminobutyric acid receptor complex at a site distinct from barbiturates. J Pharmacol Exp Ther 1989;248:960–6.
117. Majewska MD. Neurosteroids: endogenous bimodal modulators of the GAGA-A receptor: mechanism of action and physiological significance. Prog Neurobiol 1992;38:379–95.
118. Lambert JJ, Belelli D, Hill-Venning C, et al. Neurosteroids and GABA$_A$ receptor function. Trends Pharmacol Sci 1995;16:295–303.
119. Ahboucha S, Pomier-Layrargues G, Mamar O, et al. Increased levels of pregnenolone and its neuroactive metabolite allopregnenolone in autopsied brain tissue from cirrhotic patients who died in hepatic coma. Neurochem Int 2006; 49:372–8.
120. Majewska MD, Schwartz RD. Pregnenolone-sulfate: an endogenous antagonist of the gamma-aminobutyric acid receptor complex in brain? Brain Res 1987; 404:355–60.
121. Itzak Y, Norenberg MD. Attenuation of ammonia toxicity in mice by PK 11195 and pregnenolone sulphate. Neurosci Lett 1994;182:251–4.
122. Norenberg MD. Astroglial dysfunction in hepatic encephalopathy. Metab Brain Dis 1998;13:319–35.
123. Butterworth RF. The astrocytic ("peripheral-type") benzodiazepine receptor: role in the pathogenesis of portal-systemic encephalopathy. Neurochem Int 2000;36: 411–6.
124. Desjardins P, Butterworth RF. The "peripheral-type" benzodiazepine (omega 3) receptor in hyperammonemic disorders. Neurochem Int 2002;41:109–14.
125. Ahboucha S, Butterworth RF. The neurosteroid system: implication in the pathogenesis of hepatic encephalopathy. Neurochem Int 2008;52:575–87.
126. Ahboucha S. Neurosteroids and hepatic encephalopathy: an update on possible pathophysiologic mechanisms. Curr Mol Pharmacol 2011;4:1–13.

Assessment and Usefulness of Clinical Scales for Semiquantification of Overt Hepatic Encephalopathy

Maiko Sakamoto, PhD[a], William Perry, PhD[b], Robin C. Hilsabeck, PhD[c,d], Fatma Barakat, BA[e], Tarek Hassanein, MD[e,*]

KEYWORDS

- Overt hepatic encephalopathy • Clinical scales
- Neuropsychological tests • Neurophysiologic tests
- Hepatic encephalopathy assessment • HESA • WHC
- Cirrhosis

Hepatic encephalopathy (HE) represents the secondary effects of liver dysfunction on the brain. HE is a spectrum of neuropsychiatric manifestations seen in patients with liver dysfunction and portal-systemic shunting, after the exclusion of other brain diseases.[1] It affects 30% to 45% of patients with cirrhosis, and its presence and degree of progression signify poor prognosis and high mortality.[2]

Multiple mechanisms are involved in the pathophysiology of HE occurring in the presence of liver cell dysfunctions and portosystemic shunting.[3,4] The brain functions affected in patients with HE are typically categorized into 4 major clinically relevant areas.[5] These areas include consciousness, intellectual functions, personality changes, and neuromuscular manifestations.

[a] Department of Psychiatry, University of California, San Diego, 220 Dickinson Street, Suite B (MC: 8231), San Diego, CA 92103, USA
[b] Department of Psychiatry, University of California, San Diego, 200 West Arbor Drive (MC: 8218), San Diego, CA 92103, USA
[c] Department of Psychiatry, University of Texas Health Science Center at San Antonio, USA
[d] Neuropsychology Postdoctoral Residency Program, South Texas Veterans Health Care System, Psychology Service (116B), 7400 Merton Minter Boulevard, San Antonio, TX 78229, USA
[e] Southern California Liver Centers, 230 Prospect Place, Suite 220, Coronado, CA 92118, USA
* Corresponding author.
E-mail address: thassanein@livercenters.com

Clin Liver Dis 16 (2012) 27–42
doi:10.1016/j.cld.2011.12.005
1089-3261/12/$ – see front matter © 2012 Elsevier Inc. All rights reserved.

liver.theclinics.com

HE can be mild to the point that the neuropsychiatric changes are minimal and can be easily missed by physical examination and only detected by special cognitive testing. This degree of HE is currently known as covert HE (subclinical or minimal). If the HE is clinically obvious, it is termed overt HE (OHE).[6] OHE is graded depending on the degree of brain dysfunction, ranging from mild brain impairment to severe brain dysfunction and coma. Even severe states of HE and coma can vary in the degree of functional brain suppression as reflected by the Glasgow Coma Scale (GCS).[7]

HE is also classified as type A, B, or C depending on the disease state of the liver. The degree of reversibility of the neuropsychological dysfunction and the course of the dysfunction result in further classification of HE into episodic, persistent, or minimal.

The reversibility of the neuropsychological dysfunction is well documented in patients with effective therapies, recovery of liver cell function, and in patients after liver transplantation.[8] However, a significant number of patients with chronic liver disease manifest subtle neurocognitive dysfunctions related to the underlying liver disease (hepatitis C virus, nonalcoholic steatohepatitis, alcoholic liver disease) or as a result of other disease states and comorbidities, and is not related to liver cell dysfunction or portosystemic shunting.[9–14] These neurocognitive dysfunctions are always a challenge to separate from the HE seen in patients with advanced liver disease.

SCORING SYSTEMS FOR OHE

Scoring systems have been developed to assess the severity of HE, monitor patient response to therapy and intervention, and help in defining the short-term and long-term prognosis of the patient. Although most scoring systems are arbitrary, there is a continued effort to refine and standardize them.[15] The following represents the primary scoring systems used in both research and clinical practice to assess HE. Each of the systems was developed to address the lack of a well-validated, standardized approach to assessing HE.

CLINICAL SCALES
West Haven Criteria (Conn Score)

The West Haven Criteria (WHC) were among the first efforts in assessing the severity of HE. Based on a clinical examination, HE is classified into 1 of 4 grades, depending on the state of consciousness and supported by assessing other affected brain functions, including a subjective assessment of intellectual functions, personality and behavior changes, and neuromuscular manifestations (**Table 1**).[16] Although clinically simple in its use, the scale involves testing complex brain functions in a semiquantitative form. Its use gained popularity both clinically and in clinical trials. A major criticism against the WHC is its subjectivity and lack of specific definitions for the assessed dysfunctions and decreased precision in differentiating the early and late grades of HE.[17] However, it established a model for assessing the brain functions that are clinically relevant. The WHC is used clinically in a simplified form in which patients are assessed at the bedside into 4 grades (**Table 2**).[5] Grade 0 indicates absence of overt neuropsychiatric or neurologic symptoms or signs, and grade 4 indicates severe HE and coma. Its precise implementation requires up to 15 minutes, although, when used at the bedside during clinical rounds, it takes less time.[1,15]

The WHC has been used as the main scoring system in recent clinical trials evaluating new therapies for HE. In a recent study by Bass and colleagues[18] evaluating the efficacy of rifaximin in preventing relapse of HE in patients with cirrhosis who had history of overt HE, the investigators used the WHC to grade the stage of HE but failed

Table 1
Stages of hepatic encephalopathy according to the West Haven scale

Grade of Encephalopathy	State of Consciousness	Intellectual Function	Personality-Behavior	Neuromuscular Abnormalities
0 = Normal	No abnormality	No abnormality	No abnormality	No abnormality
1 = Mild impairment	Inverted sleep pattern Insomnia/ hypersomnia	Impaired computations: complex Short attention span	Euphoria Depression Irritability	Tremor Impaired concentration Asterixis, grade 1
2 = Moderate impairment	Slow responses Lethargy	Impaired computations: simple Amnesia for recent events Loss of time	Personality changes Anxiety Apathy/ inappropriate behavior	Asterixis, grades 2 and 3 Slurred speech Hyperactive reflexes Ataxia
3 = Severe impairment	Somnolence/ semistupor Confusion	Inability to compute Loss of place	Bizarre behavior Paranoia Anger/rage	Clonus/rigidity Nystagmus Babinski
4 = Coma	Stupor Unconscious	No intellect	None	Coma Dilated pupils Opisthotonus

From Blei AT. Hepatic encephalopathy. In: Kaplowitz N, editor. Liver and biliary diseases, 2nd ed. Baltimore (MD): Williams & Wilkins; 1996. p. 623; with permission.

to mention that the grading was reached by implementing the Hepatic Encephalopathy Scoring Algorithm (HESA).

HESA

The HESA[17] was developed to capitalize on the strengths of the WHC but improve on the WHC by introducing objective indicators of cognitive impairment. The HESA combines the clinical examination with neuropsychological tests in an effort to improve objectivity and increase sensitivity when determining HE grade. The HESA was designed to minimize effects of education; consequently, in most cases age

Table 2
Stages of HE according to the West Haven scale

Grade	Neurologic Manifestations
0	No alteration in consciousness, intellectual function, personality, or behavior
1	Trivial lack of awareness, euphoria or anxiety, shortened attention span, impaired performance of addition
2	Lethargy or apathy, minimal disorientation for time or place, subtle personality change, inappropriate behavior, impaired performance of subtraction
3	Somnolence to semistupor but responsive to verbal stimuli, confusion; gross disorientation
4	Coma; no response to verbal or noxious stimuli

From Conn HO, Leevy CM, Vlahcevic ZR, et al. Comparison of lactulose and neomycin in the treatment of chronic portal-systemic encephalopathy. A double blind controlled trial. Gastroenterology 1977;72(4 Pt 1):575; with permission.

and education transformation is not required. It relies mostly on findings from the clinical examination in the more severe grades for which neuropsychological testing is not possible (eg, grades 4 and 3), and more heavily on objective cognitive testing in the lower grades in which dysfunction may be subtle and less obvious on clinical examination (eg, grades 2 and 1) (**Table 3**). The HESA also provides both continuous and categorical distinctions. The neuropsychological tasks were carefully chosen based on the following criteria: (1) well validated and standardized, (2) brief, and (3) easy to administer and score. With great consideration, neuropsychological measures of the HESA include the following cognitive tasks: orientation, mental control, list learning, computations, digit span, and visuoconstruction, as well as depression and anxiety ratings. Based on a decision tree considering both clinical and neuropsychological outcomes, an HE severity score is determined.

The HESA has 6 alternate forms and is one of the few HE grading tools that assesses all severity levels of HE, making it a good choice for tracking changes over time, and initial findings indicate that it is more sensitive than the WHC.[17] In a pivotal multicenter, multinational, placebo-controlled clinical trial examining the efficacy of rifaximin for

Table 3
HESA

Time			:		24 Hour Clock		

4	○No eyes opening	○No verbal/voice response
	○No reaction to simple commands	

All applicable ⇒ Grade 4 ○   otherwise continue examination

3	○Somnolence ○Confusion ○Disoriented to place
	○Bizarre Behavior / Anger/Rage ○Clonus/Rigidity /Nysatgmus / Babinsky
	□Mental Control = 0

3 or more applicable ⇒ Grade 3 ○   otherwise continue examination

2	○Lethargy ○Loss of time ○Slurred Speech
	○Hyperactive Reflexes ○Inappropriate Behavior
	□ Slow Responses □ Amnesia of recent events
	□ Anxiety □ Impaired Simple Computations

2 or more ○and 3 or more □ applicable ⇒ Grade 2 ○ otherwise continue

1	○Sleep disorder / Impaired Sleep Pattern ○Tremor
	□ Impaired complex computations □ Shortened attention span
	□ Impaired Construction ability □ Euphoria or Depression

4 or more applicable ⇒ Grade 1 ○   otherwise Grade 0

HE Grade	|_|

NOTE: ○indicates symptoms assessed using clinical judgment and □ indicates symptoms assessed using neuropsychological measures.

Copyright © 2006 The Regents of the University of California

From Hassanein TI, Hilsabeck RC, Perry W. Introduction to the Hepatic Encephalopathy Scoring Algorithm (HESA). Dig Dis Sci 2008;53(2):530; with permission.

maintenance of remission from HE, the HESA was used to ensure objectivity of WHC scores and was found to have good precision in differentiating grades 0, 1, and 2 (**Table 4**).[19] There was no significant variability within or among study sites, indicating good inter-rater reliability of the HESA, consistent with prior findings.[20] Although more validation of the HESA is needed, it is a viable option for clinical trials because the neuropsychological tests used are well known and widely available. It has been suggested that the HESA may be useful in differentiating patients with end-stage liver disease who are cognitively intact versus those people with minimal HE who are at risk for developing OHE. Hassanein and colleagues[17] showed that some patients rated as grade 0 according to the WHC exhibited cognitive indicators of impairment, indicating grade 1.

The HESA has also been successfully used to objectively assess cognitive changes during extracorporeal albumin dialysis (ECAD) in patients with cirrhosis and severe encephalopathy (grades 3 and 4). In a study of 597 evaluations in patients randomized to ECAD plus standard medical therapy or the latter only, it was shown that the HESA was useful in evaluating clinical changes in patients with severe HE.

Consequently the HESA provides a single measurement that can encompass the broad spectrum of neurologic and clinical manifestations of HE. Like the WHC, it is simple and time efficient and sensitive to subtle brain changes but offers a more objective approach, which should yield greater reliability across the spectrum of HE.

Clinical Hepatic Encephalopathy Staging Scale

The Clinical Hepatic Encephalopathy Staging Scale (CHESS)[20] was designed to monitor the severity of HE on a scale from 0 (low) to 9 (high). This score is based on observations of 9 manifestations of HE that are categorized into dichotomous groups

Table 4
HESA confirmation of WHC scoring in rifaximin trial

HESA Category	HESA Indicator	Conn Score = 0 N = 129	Conn Score = 1 N = 43	Conn Score = 2 N = 0	P Value Conn 0 vs 1
		Patients, n (%)			
Clinical	Sleep disorder/ impaired sleep pattern	32 (25)	27 (63)	—	<.0001
Clinical	Tremor	17 (13)	21 (49)	—	<.0001
Clinical	Inappropriate/bizarre behavior	0	0	—	—
Clinical	Disorientation to place	0	0	—	—
Neuropsychological	Amnesia of recent events	64 (50)	32 (74)	—	.0047
Neuropsychological	Impaired simple computations	4 (3)	6 (14)	—	.0167
Neuropsychological	Impaired complex computations	31 (24)	18 (42)	—	.0320
Neuropsychological	Depression	17 (13)	13 (30)	—	.0186

Note: This table was presented at the Food and Drug Administration, Center for Drug Evaluation and Research (CDER) Meeting of the Gastrointestinal Drugs Advisory Committee (GIDAC) on February 23, 2010.

From Forbes WP. Efficacy of rifaximin for treatment of hepatic encephalopathy. Xifaxan (rifaximin) tablets 550 mg for hepatic encephalopathy 2010. Available at: www.fda.gov/downloads/AdvisoryCommittees/./UCM203248.pdf; with permission.

(**Table 5**). The determination of presence/absence of each manifestation is clear enough that the CHESS can be administered by health care providers without specialized training in HE. Factor analysis supported 2 factors, mild and severe HE, which is in line with recent calls to classify HE into more clinically meaningful categories rather than trying to make fine-grained differentiations among grades 0 to 4. The CHESS should be augmented with the GCS when refined discrimination of more severe HE is desired.[20]

GCS

The GCS is a ubiquitous neurologic scoring system devised in 1974 for bedside assessment of consciousness.[7] It is currently used as a universal standard for assessment of mental status in patients with traumatic brain injury. It scores eye opening, verbal responses, and motor responses. The highest possible score is 15 and the lowest is 3. The GCS score is helpful in assessing patients with severe HE (grades III and IV) but is not useful when assessing early grades (<I, I, II). It correlates strongly with the HESA ($r = 0.85$) and with CHESS ($r = 0.79$).[20,21] The limitation of using GCS is the significant overlap in the range of GCS scores among all grades of HE (**Table 6**). However, it is suggested that it could help in making fine discriminations in severe HE.[20,21]

NEUROPSYCHOLOGICAL TESTS
Portosystemic Encephalopathy Index

The Portosystemic Encephalopathy Index (PSEI) was first introduced by Conn and colleagues[5] and combines neuropsychological parameters (Trail-making Test [TMT]),

Table 5 CHESS	
1. Does the patient know which month he/she is in (i.e.: January, February)?	
0. Yes.	1. No, or he/she does not talk.
2. Does the patient know which day of the week he/she is in (i.e.: Thursday, Friday, Sunday…)?	
0. Yes.	1. No, or he/she does not talk.
3. Can he/she count backwards from 10 to 1 without making mistakes or stopping?	
0. Yes.	1. No, or he/she does not talk.
If asked to do so, does he/she raise his/her arms?	
0. Yes.	1. No.
5. Does he/she understand what you are saying to him/her? (based on the answers to questions 1 to 4)	
0. Yes.	1. No, or he/she does not talk.
6. Is the patient awake and alert?	
0. Yes.	1. No, he/she is sleepy or fast asleep.
7. Is the patient fast asleep, and is it difficult to wake him/her up?	
0. Yes.	1. No.
8. Can he/she talk?	
0. Yes.	1. He/she does not talk.
9. Can he/she talk correctly? In other words, can you understand everything he/she says, and he/she doesn't stammer?	
0. Yes.	1. No, he/she does not talk or does not talk correctly.

From Ortiz M, Cordoba J, Doval E, et al. Development of a clinical hepatic encephalopathy staging scale. Aliment Pharmacol Ther 2007;26(6):S1; with permission.

Table 6 GCS score by HE grade determined by HESA	
Grade of HE	Median GCS Score (Range of Scores)
IV	3 (3–12)
III	11 (3–15)
II	14 (3–15)
I	15 (11–15)
<1	15 (11–15)

GCS scores range from 3 (lowest score) to 15 (highest score).
Data from Hassanein T, Blei AT, Perry W, et al. Performance of the hepatic encephalopathy scoring algorithm in a clinical trial of patients with cirrhosis and severe hepatic encephalopathy. Am J Gastroenterol 2009;104(6):1392–400.

neurophysiologic (electroencephalogram [EEG]) and biochemical (arterial ammonia) tests, clinical assessment of mental status, and degree of asterixis to diagnose HE. The PSEI has been calculated several ways, which are often used as a formula: 3 × mental state score + TMT score + asterixis score + ammonia score.[22] The TMT is a test of visual attention, psychomotor speed, and mental switching that requires a subject to connect dots of consecutive targets. There are 2 parts to the test. The first is TMT-A, in which the targets are all numbers, and the second is TMT-B, in which the subject alternates between numbers and letters. The subject is required to complete each part as quickly as possible. The total time to completion and number of errors are used as performance indicators. The TMT is also known as the number connection test in the liver disease literature and is widely regarded as a sensitive psychometric measure for the assessment of early HE. Early use of the test did not take into account differences in performance based on important factors such as age and educational level; however, in recent studies, the patient's performance has been evaluated based on normative data corrected for age and level of education to reduce the number of false-positive classification errors. Furthermore, neuropsychological tests are subject to practice effects such that improvement occurs by virtue of prior exposure. To minimize practice effects, it is important to have alternate forms of equal difficulty. Regarding the biochemical markers of the PSEI some have argued that ammonia levels should not be used. Ferenci and colleagues[23] suggested that arterial ammonia levels are arbitrary and can lead to spurious results limiting the use of the PSEI. Although the EEG is considered to be an objective gold standard in the detection of HE, Amodio and colleagues[24–27] point out that its interpretation may be biased by interobserver variability.[4] Consequently, members of the Working Party at the 11th World Congresses of Gastroenterology, Vienna, 1998 concluded, "In episodic (acute) encephalopathy, the PSE index has not been determined to be superior to clinical grading. Its shortcomings limit its use for the quantification of HE in clinical studies of chronic encephalopathy."[23]

Psychometric Hepatic Encephalopathy Score and Portosystemic Encephalopathy Syndrome Test

The Psychometric Hepatic Encephalopathy Score (PHES) was standardized and validated by Weissenborn and colleagues[28] as an assessment tool of minimal HE (MHE). The PHES first comprised 7 tests: the line tracing test (LTT), serial dotting test (SDT), digit symbol test (DST), number connection test A and B (NCT A and B), digit span test (DST), and the canceling *d*-test.[29] However, the desire for a shorter battery and poor sensitivity of some of the tests led to the introduction of the revised battery called the

Portosystemic Encephalopathy (PSE) Syndrome Test, which included the NCT A and B, LTT, SDT, and DST only.[24,28] When interpreting the PHES and PSE Syndrome Test, like other neuropsychological measures, it is important to consider the influence of age, sex, education, and cultural differences on test performance. The proper use of these measures has resulted in a short, objective, reliable means of assessing MHE at the bedside. The test administration is approximately 10 to 15 minutes. Regarding scoring, test results within 1 standard deviation (SD) were assigned a score of 0, those between 1 and 2 SD less than the mean were assigned a score of −1, those between 2 and 3 SD less than the mean were assigned a −2, and those beyond 3 SD less than the mean were assigned a score of −3. Test results better than 1 SD more than the mean were assigned a score of +1. A total score ranges from −18 to +6. Using a cut point of −4, sensitivity and specificity of the PHES compared with the standard method of determining HE grade were 96% and 100%, respectively. Standard normative data of the PHES have been developed in German,[28,30] Spanish,[31,32] Italian,[24] and Mexican.[33] Thus, the PHES is predominantly used for detecting minimal HE in Europe.

Repeatable Battery for the Assessment of Neuropsychological Status

The Repeatable Battery for the Assessment of Neuropsychological Status (RBANS)[34] is a brief (ie, 20–25 minutes) paper-and-pencil battery designed to screen for cognitive impairment. It yields a summary score of global cognitive functioning based on 5 domain scores measuring language, visuoperception, attention, immediate memory, and delayed memory. It has 4 alternate forms and has been translated into at least 20 languages. Although a few studies have now confirmed its usefulness in characterizing cognitive impairment in liver transplant candidates[35–37] and the International Society for Hepatic Encephalopathy and Nitrogen Metabolism (ISHEN) recommended it for use in patients at risk for developing minimal HE,[38] there are limited data to support its use in patients with OHE. Many patients with grade 2 HE can not complete the RBANS because of difficulty attending to test procedures and/or tolerating the testing process, and patients in grades 3 and 4 HE definitely are not able to because the degree of impaired consciousness (ie, somnolence in grade 3 and coma in grade 4) interferes with their ability to attend to, and/or understand, task instructions for more than a few seconds (in grade 3), if at all (in grade 4).

Critical Flicker Frequency

Critical flicker frequency (CFF) is a neuropsychological/neurophysiologic technique that assesses the cerebral cortex function. It has been used to detect a range of neuropsychological abnormalities from visual signal processing to cognitive functions. Thus, its usefulness has been established in a variety of fields including neurology, psychiatry, and ophthalmology.[32,39,40] In recent studies, the CFF has been proposed as an objective measure for grading HE[41] as well as using it as a tool for assessing cirrhotic patients' recovery from sedation after endoscopy, a marker of HE in patients undergoing transjugular intrahepatic portosystemic shunt as well as differentiating between fatigue and HE in patients with primary biliary cirrhosis.[42–44]

The CFF is a portable analyzer, with head-mounted goggles into which the patient is asked to look. The controller evokes an intrafoveal light stimulus, red light pulses at preconfigured wavelength, luminance, luminous intensity, and a specified ratio between the visual impulse and the interval starting from a high frequency of 60 Hz and being gradually reduced. At this high frequency, the light appears steady (fused). The light pulse frequency is gradually decreased, which gives the impression that the light is flickering/pulsating. The patient is asked to register when this change happens by pressing a handgrip button, and this determines the CFF threshold. The test is repeated about 8 to 10 times and the average CFF threshold is calculated. The test takes about 15 to 20 minutes to complete.[39–41]

There is no consensus on the cutoff for an abnormal CFF.[1] Furthermore, studies have focused on minimal HE. Most published studies agree that the sensitivity and specificity of CFF diagnosing MHE is 80% and 65% respectively.[41] A CFF less than 39 Hz represented the borderline between HE 0 and HE 1, not the cutoff for MHE diagnosis, whereas a CFF less than 38 Hz was used as an artificial borderline for predicting further bouts of HE 1. Romero-Gomez and colleagues[32] found that "CFF together with Child-Pugh class predicts the development of [HE 1–2] in follow-up."

The CFF is supposed to be a simple, easy-to-use, and reliable tool that is independent of education, gender, age, and literacy. However, further validation and standardization studies are needed to determine its use and applicability in differentiating between HE grades 0 and 1. Although current data indicate the predictability of OHE, this has mostly been defined as HE grade 1 and, in some studies, as HE 2. Therefore, CFF has not been established as a diagnostic tool in overt HE.

Continuous Reaction Time

Continuous reaction times (CRT) were more widely used in the past as a sensitive measure for detecting brain dysfunctions of various origins (organic vs metabolic). In this test, the patient is asked to press a button, with their dominant hand, as fast as possible when exposed to a series of auditory signals from earphones (500 Hz, 90dB). The signals are delivered by a tape recorder triggered via a computer and the reaction times are recorded on punched tape. The signals are presented at random intervals of 2 to 6 seconds, 15 signals per minutes. There is a 2-minute run-in period followed by a 10-minute test period that consists of 150 signals. If the patient does not respond to the stimulus within 2 seconds, it is registered as no response.[40,45]

All published studies on CRT focused on patients with cirrhosis and HE grades 0 to 2. Their findings indicated that the 90 percentile (0.225 seconds) best discriminated between controls and patients with HE with 82% of patients with HE correctly classified.[45,46] In addition, the percentile ratio between the 50 percentile and the difference between the 10 and 90 percentile was able to differentiate the best between patients with HE and patients with brain damage.[45,46]

Although auditory CRT is a reliable measure, suitable for serial assessment, and its sensitivity and specificity in HE are 0.97 and 0.64 respectively, it is not practical, applicable, or useful in diagnosing OHE. One of its main limitations is its use in patients with hearing problems. There have been other variations of CRT in which, in addition to measuring the auditory reaction time, the speed of reaction to light (visual) and choice stimuli were introduced and measured. Nevertheless, the same conclusion is reached; that is, CRT might be considered a diagnostic tool in MHE, but not in OHE.[47]

Inhibitory Control Test

The Inhibitory Control Test (ICT) is a computerized test measuring attention and response inhibition. This test has been used to detect attention deficits in persons with traumatic brain injury, schizophrenia, and attention-deficit/hyperactivity disorder. Bajaj and colleagues[48] extended the use of the test to identify individuals with MHE. The ICT is similar to other go-no-go or continuous performance tests (CPT) and assesses sustained attention as well as the ability to inhibit responses to nontargets. It consists of a continuous stream of letters presented on a computer screen every 500 milliseconds. The examinee is required to respond when certain alternating patterns involving the letters X and Y (ie, targets) are presented. Examinees must be careful not to respond when nontarget presentations of the letters X and Y (ie, lures) appear. A total of 212 targets and 40 lures, along with numerous extraneous letters, are presented in one 15-minute administration, which includes 1 training session and 6 tests. The percentage of targets and lures responded to, as well as reaction time, are recorded. Bajaj and colleagues[48,49] showed that a cut point of more than 5 lures yielded a 90% classification accuracy for the diagnosis of MHE, and test-retest reliability was 90 with an approximately 2-month interval. However, another study reported that lures alone were not sensitive in detecting MHE; target accuracy and lures weighted by target accuracy showed better discriminating values between healthy controls and MHE plus individuals.[25] The ICT has been also used in driving studies, which showed that ICT performance was significantly associated with driving simulator performance and traffic accidents.[49,50] CPT measures like the ICT have gained prominence in detecting cognitive-based attention and inhibitory problems but deficits on the ICT are not necessarily specific to any particular disorder. Furthermore, like other neuropsychological measures, the ICT is influenced by prior exposure.[25] Although the ICT is a promising instrument, further research is needed to support its use as a tool to diagnose MHE.

Scan Test

Another neuropsychological measure that is based on reaction time and the Sternberg paradigm is the scan test. It is a computerized digit recognizing task in which a series of 36 randomly sorted pairs of numbers are displayed on a computer screen for 3 seconds each. Subjects are then asked to tap either 1 or 3 on the keyboard, indicating whether they had recognized a common digit in the pair of numbers. Thus, in addition to measuring the mean reaction time, this test measures the percentage of errors in recognizing whether there is at least 1 common digit between pairs of number (2–4 digits) subsequently displayed on the screen. Age and education z scores are computed and a z score of 2 or more standard deviations less than the reference value indicates a failed test.[26]

The scan test has been used in several studies in cirrhotic patients with and without minimal HE. The consensus has been that it is of value in detecting the neuropsychological impairment caused by cirrhosis. About 50% of cirrhotic patients performed poorly on the scan test. Furthermore, patients who had history of OHE performed significantly worse than those who never had a bout of OHE. Taking it a step further, in the most recent published study on scan tests, Amodio and colleagues[26] found that, among various types of psychometric tests such as the Trail-making Tests and Symbol Digit Modality Tests, the scan test was the most closely related to central brain atrophy. This is in line with the way the scan test "reflects prefrontal cortex functioning… which, in turn, is influenced by basal nuclei."[26]

Although this neuropsychological measure assesses cognitive domains that have been proved to be impaired in MHE, it is of minimal use as a diagnostic measure in patients with OHE, especially grades 3 and 4, primarily because of its computerized application. However, the performance of cirrhotic patients without history of OHE on the scan test illustrates the impact and damage caused by having any episode of OHE in the past, which emphasizes the seriousness of OHE.

NEUROPHYSIOLOGIC TESTS
Magnetic Resonance Imaging

On magnetic resonance imaging (MRI), typical findings in HE include hyperintensities in the globus pallidus on T1-weighted images thought to be caused by manganese accumulation and white matter abnormalities on fast fluid-attenuated inversion recovery sequences (FLAIR) and diffusion-weighted images (DWI) secondary to edema.[51]

Proton Magnetic Resonance Spectroscopy

The most common findings in HE when using proton magnetic resonance spectroscopy (^{1}H MRS) are increased glutamine/glutamate peaks accompanied by decreased myoinositol and choline caused by astrocyte swelling and brain edema.[51,52]

EEG and Evoked Potentials

It has been suggested that electrophysiologic testing such as quantitative EEG analysis and evoked potentials (EPs) can be useful for the diagnosis of HE. EEG is the technique of recording spontaneous electrical brain activity from the scalp and correlating it with the underlying brain function. It has been widely proposed that electrophysiologic methods are more objective for the detection of HE than bedside examination.[53,54] In mild HE, the increase in confusion is associated with the initial EEG tracings that reveal posterior dominant α rhythm slowing, which is typically followed by a gradual appearance of θ and δ waves. As the HE progresses into more severe states, the EEG tracings are characterized by high-amplitude irregular δ activity. EEG tracings can also contain a suppression-burst pattern consisting of regular alternation between low-amplitude and high-amplitude activity. Although EEG is a robust tool, there is interobserver variability leading some to suggest a lack of objectivity.[27] One alternative approach is spectral EEG or a computerized analysis of the frequency distribution in the EEG. Amodio and colleagues[27] reported that spectral analysis EEG was more reliable than visual EEG reading and provided an objective staging of HE. They also reported that, although computerized spectral EEG classification of HE could improve the repeatability of EEG assessment of normal and clearly altered EEG tracings, the grading of mild HE needs further improvements before it could be recommended for clinical practice.[27]

Another specialized psychophysiologic approach is that of EPs, which are computed by measuring the latency between the onset of a stimulus and the brain's detection of the stimulus as observed through EEG recording. EPs can be delivered through auditory, visual, or somatosensory modalities and require active patient cooperation. Consequently, the use of EPs is limited in patients with OHE. The P300 is an event-related potential that is elicited by oddball or low-probability target items interspersed among high-probability nonstimuli. In response to the oddball stimuli, the brain shows an EEG recognition response at approximately 300 to 600 milliseconds. A delay response greater than 300 milliseconds indicates brain impairment. Both auditory and visual P300 have been shown to have diagnostic potential in mild HE[55] but are nonspecific to HE and not recommended because of inconsistent results.

In general, electrophysiologic techniques have great promise in diagnosing and staging HE; however, the lack of a precise definition of what constitutes the MHE and the absence of clear cutoffs and guidelines for the sensitivity and specificity of these techniques limit their clinical usefulness. Furthermore, EEG equipment is expensive, requires specialized settings, and is prone to subjective interpretation. Some researchers suggest that expensive equipment, low sensitivity, and the lack of accompanying behavioral information are drawbacks of these methods.[56,57]

Bispectral Index

According to the Consensus Statement of the 1998 World Congress of Gastroenterology, a quantitative neurophysiologic measure such as EEG should be used whenever possible.[23] However, EEG is time consuming, expensive, and not readily available. A quick and easy-to-use bispectral index (BIS) monitor was designed to monitor the effects of anesthetic/sedative drugs and has been approved for such use by the US Food and Drug Administration in 1996.[58] The BIS monitoring system is designed to monitor the hypnotic state of the brain based on acquisition and processing of EEG signals. By placing a sensor strip on the patient's forehead, the BIS retrieves the signal. The total time to complete the procedure is approximately 10 minutes.

The BIS system processes raw EEG signals to produce a single number, called the BIS, which correlates with the patient's level of consciousness/hypnosis. The index ranges from 0 to 100, with 100 indicating a fully awake state; 70 to 60 indicating light hypnotic effects; 60 to 40 indicating moderate hypnotic effects; and less than 40, deep hypnotic effect.[58] The BIS is the weighted sum of 3 subparameters: relative β ratio, (BetaRatio) a frequency domain feature; relative synchrony of fast and slow wave, (SynchFastSlow) a bispectral domain feature; and burst suppression ratio, a time domain feature.[59]

Bispectral analysis has been the focus of several studies in patients with liver disease. Most of the studies used BIS in monitoring consciousness before, during, and after liver transplant with a closer examination of the type of transplant and reason for transplant. However, to date, there has been 1 published study with the main objective of assessing the sensitivity and specificity of BIS in classifying OHE.[59]

Dahaba and colleagues[59] found that, with a high discriminative power, BIS could be used as a diagnostic tool in differentiating between the different HE grades because of its ability to accurately detect and display the graduated increase in the β power.[59] BIS had a slightly higher discriminative power for HE grades 3 and 4. In addition, BIS maintained its high discriminative power across time and was independent of inter-rater and intra-rater variability. A BIS cutoff value of 95 indicated West Haven HE grade 1, 85 corresponded with an HE grade 2, 70 was HE grade 3, and 55 indicated HE grade 4.[59]

In summary, in OHE, BIS is a simple, inexpensive, objective, and real-time measure of consciousness independent of cause, ammonia levels, Child-Pugh score, MELD score, and rater variability. BIS correlates well with West Haven grade and GCS, and, in an intensive care unit setting, can predict the patient's responses such as timing of opening the eyes, movement, and the possibility of brain death. However, caution is warranted when interpreting its results in the presence of electromyogram (EMG) activity,[58,59] and its use needs further validations in assessing grades of HE.

SUMMARY

Hepatic encephalopathy (also called portosystematic encephalopathy) is a serious complication of advanced liver disease and manifests as neuropsychiatric abnormalities such as altered levels of consciousness, cognitive impairment, confusion, and mood abnormalities. When HE is clinically obvious, it is termed OHE. Assessing the severity of HE is critical because it is associated with high mortality and poor prognosis, but it is often reversible with effective therapy. This article discusses the major methods for grading HE, including those methods that rely on clinical ratings, neuropsychological tests, and neurophysiologic measures, and addresses some of the limitations in each of the methods. Recently, there has been a great effort to develop valid and reliable HE assessment tools. Although there continues to be question as to the best method to reliably assess the full spectrum of neuropsychiatric abnormalities associated with HE, the field is moving closer to developing a sensitive measure. It is essential for clinicians to closely monitor the patient with HE. A combination of psychometric and electrophysiologic tests provides one option to detect HE. When the inclusion of electrophysiology is not feasible, using an objective psychometric measure, such as the HESA, holds promise as a quick and portable assessment that has been translated into several languages and has alternate forms. The HESA is a sensitive multimethod approach to grading HE that can allow for a more objective comparison of results across time. Furthermore, although the relationship between electrophysiology measures and functional assessment (everyday function) has yet to be established, psychometric measures have been shown to have direct relevance to activities of daily living[60] and quality of life.[61] Well-designed studies are still needed to characterize each of the methods used to assess HE and to compare the results with established efficacy parameters in the treatment of HE.

REFERENCES

1. Prakash R, Mullen KD. Mechanisms, diagnosis and management of hepatic encephalopathy. Nat Rev Gastroenterol Hepatol 2010;7(9):515–25.
2. Albrecht J. Hepatic encephalopathy in our genes? Ann Intern Med 2010;153(5): 335–6.
3. Bismuth M, Funakoshi N, Cadranel J, et al. Hepatic encephalopathy: from pathophysiology to therapeutic management. Eur J Gastroenterol Hepatol 2001;23(1): 8–22.
4. Cordoba J, Minguez B. Hepatic encephalopathy. Semin Liver Dis 2008;28(1): 70–80.
5. Conn HO, Leevy CM, Vlahcevic ZR, et al. Comparison of lactulose and neomycin in the treatment of chronic portal-systemic encephalopathy. A double blind controlled trial. Gastroenterology 1977;72(4 Pt 1):573–83.
6. Frederick RT. Current concepts in the pathophysiology and management of hepatic encephalopathy. Gestroenterol Hepatol 2001;7:222–33.
7. Treasdale G, Jennett B. Assessment of coma and impaired consciousness: a practical scale. Lancet 1974;304:81–4.
8. Teperman LW, Peyregne VP. Considerations on the impact of hepatic encephalopathy treatments in the pretransplant setting. Transplantation 2010;89(7):771–8.
9. Rovira A, Cordoba J, Sanpedro F, et al. Normalization of T2 signal abnormalities in hemispheric white matter with liver transplant. Neurology 2002;59(3):335–41.
10. Garcia-Martinez R, Rovira A, Alonso J, et al. Hepatic encephalopathy is associated with posttransplant cognitive function and brain volume. Liver Transpl 2011;17(1):38–46.
11. Hilsabeck RC, Perry W, Hassanein TI. Neuropsychological impairment in patients with chronic hepatitis C. Hepatology 2002;35(2):440–6.
12. Forton DM, Thomas HC, Murphy CA, et al. Hepatitis C and cognitive impairment in a cohort of patients with mild liver disease. Hepatology 2002;35(2):433–9.
13. Saner FH, Nadalin S, Radtke A, et al. Liver transplantation and neurological side effects. Metab Brain Dis 2009;24(1):183–7.
14. McAndrews MP, Farcnik K, Carlen P, et al. Prevalence and significance of neurocognitive dysfunction in hepatitis C in the absence of correlated risk factors. Hepatology 2005;41(4):801–8.
15. Cordoba J. New assessment of hepatic encephalopathy. J Hepatol 2011;54(5): 1030–40.
16. Blei AT. Hepatic encephalopathy. In: Kaplowitz N, editor. Liver and biliary diseases. 2nd edition. Baltimore (MD): Williams & Wilkins; 1996. p. 623.
17. Hassanein TI, Hilsabeck RC, Perry W. Introduction to the Hepatic Encephalopathy Scoring Algorithm (HESA). Dig Dis Sci 2008;53(2):529–38.

18. Bass NM, Mullen KD, Sanyal A, et al. Rifaximin treatment in hepatic encephalopathy. N Engl J Med 2010;362(12):1071–81.
19. Forbes WP. Efficacy of rifaximin for treatment of hepatic encephalopathy. Xifaxan® (rifaximin) Tablets 550 mg for hepatic encephalopathy 2010. Available at: www.fda.gov/downloads/AdvisoryCommittees/./UCM203248.pdf. Accessed September 22, 2011.
20. Ortiz M, Cordoba J, Doval E, et al. Development of a clinical hepatic encephalopathy staging scale. Aliment Pharmacol Ther 2007;26(6):859–67.
21. Hassanein T, Blei AT, Perry W, et al. Performance of the hepatic encephalopathy scoring algorithm in a clinical trial of patients with cirrhosis and severe hepatic encephalopathy. Am J Gastroenterol 2009;104(6):1392–400.
22. Edwin N, Peter JV, John G, et al. Relationship between clock and star drawing and the degree of hepatic encephalopathy. Postgrad Med J 2011;87(1031): 605–11.
23. Ferenci P, Lockwood A, Mullen KD, et al. Hepatic encephalopathy - definition, nomenclature, diagnosis, and quantification: final report of the working party at the 11th World Congresses of Gastroenterology, Vienna, 1998. Hepatology 2002;35(3):716–21.
24. Amodio P, Campagna F, Olianas S, et al. Detection of minimal hepatic encephalopathy: normalization and optimization of the Psychometric Hepatic Encephalopathy Score. A neuropsychological and quantified EEG study. J Hepatol 2008; 49(3):346–53.
25. Amodio P, Ridola L, Schiff S, et al. Improving the inhibitory control task to detect minimal hepatic encephalopathy. Gastroenterology 2010;139(2):510–8, 518. e511–12.
26. Amodio P, Pellegrini A, Amista P, et al. Neuropsychological-neurophysiological alterations and brain atrophy in cirrhotic patients. Metab Brain Dis 2003;18(1): 63–78.
27. Amodio P, Pellegrini A, Ubiali E, et al. The EEG assessment of low-grade hepatic encephalopathy: comparison of an artificial neural network-expert system (ANNES) based evaluation with visual EEG readings and EEG spectral analysis. Clin Neurophysiol 2006;117(10):2243–51.
28. Weissenborn K, Ennen JC, Schomerus H, et al. Neuropsychological characterization of hepatic encephalopathy. J Hepatol 2001;34(5):768–73.
29. Weissenborn K, Ennen J, Ruckert N, et al. The PSE test: an attempt to standardize neuropsychological assessment of latent portosystemic encephalopathy (PSE). In: Record CO, Al Mardini H, editors. Advances in hepatic encephalopathy and metabolism in liver disease. Newcastle upon Tyne (United Kingdom): Medical Faculty of the University of Newcastle upon Tyne; 1997. p. 489–94.
30. Schomerus H, Hamster W. Neuropsychological aspects of portal-systemic encephalopathy. Metab Brain Dis 1998;13(4):361–77.
31. Romero-Gomez M, Cordoba J, Jover R, et al. Tablas de normalidad de la poblacion espanola para los tests psicometricos utilizados en el diagnostico de la encefalopatia hepatica minima. Med Clin 2006;127:246–9.
32. Romero-Gomez M, Cordoba J, Jover R, et al. Value of the critical flicker frequency in patients with minimal hepatic encephalopathy. Hepatology 2007;45(4):879–85.
33. Duarte-Rojo A, Estradas J, Hernandez-Ramos R, et al. Validation of the Psychometric Hepatic Encephalopathy Score (PHES) for identifying patients with minimal hepatic encephalopathy. Dig Dis Sci 2011;56(10):3014–23.
34. Randolph C. Repeatable battery for the assessment of neuropsychological status manual. San Antonio (TX): Psychological Corporation; 1998.

35. Sorrell JH, Zolnikov BJ, Sharma A, et al. Cognitive impairment in people diagnosed with end-stage liver disease evaluated for liver transplantation. Psychiatry Clin Neurosci 2006;60(2):174–81.
36. Mooney S, Hasssanein TI, Hilsabeck RC, et al. Utility of the Repeatable Battery for the Assessment of Neuropsychological Status (RBANS) in patients with end-stage liver disease awaiting liver transplant. Arch Clin Neuropsychol 2007; 22(2):175–86.
37. Meyer T, Eshelman A, Abouljoud M. Neuropsychological changes in a large sample of liver transplant candidates. Transplant Proc 2006;38(10):3559–60.
38. Randolph C, Hilsabeck R, Kato A, et al. Neuropsychological assessment of hepatic encephalopathy: ISHEN practice guidelines. Liver Int 2009;29(5): 629–35.
39. Wunsch E, Post M, Gutkowski K, et al. Critical flicker frequency fails to disclose brain dysfunction in patients with primary biliary cirrhosis. Dig Liver Dis 2010; 42(11):818–21.
40. Lauridsen MM, Jepsen P, Vilstrup H. Critical flicker frequency and continuous reaction times for the diagnosis of minimal hepatic encephalopathy: a comparative study of 154 patients with liver disease. Metab Brain Dis 2011;26(2): 135–9.
41. Sharma P, Sharma BC, Sarin SK. Critical flicker frequency for diagnosis and assessment of recovery from minimal hepatic encephalopathy in patients with cirrhosis. Hepatobiliary Pancreat Dis Int 2010;9(1):27–32.
42. Sharma P, Singh S, Sharma BC, et al. Propofol sedation during endoscopy in patients with cirrhosis, and utility of psychometric tests and critical flicker frequency in assessment of recovery from sedation. Endoscopy 2011;43(5): 400–5.
43. Biecker E, Hausdorfer I, Grunhage F, et al. Critical flicker frequency as a marker of hepatic encephalopathy in patients before and after transjugular intrahepatic portosystemic shunt. Digestion 2011;83(1–2):24–31.
44. Kircheis G, Bode JG, Hilger N, et al. Diagnostic and prognostic values of critical flicker frequency determination as new diagnostic tool for objective HE evaluation in patients undergoing TIPS implantation. Eur J Gastroenterol Hepatol 2009; 21(12):1383–94.
45. Elsass P, Christensen SE, Jorgensen F, et al. Number connection test and continuous reaction times in assessment of organic and metabolic encephalopathy: a comparative study. Acta Pharmacol Toxicol (Copenh) 1984;54(2):115–9.
46. Elsass P, Christensen SE, Mortensen EL, et al. Discrimination between organic and hepatic encephalopathy by means of continuous reaction times. Liver 1985;5(1):29–34.
47. Moore JW, Dunk AA, Crawford JR, et al. Neuropsychological deficits and morphological MRI brain scan abnormalities in apparently healthy non-encephalopathic patients with cirrhosis. A controlled study. J Hepatol 1989;9(3):319–25.
48. Bajaj JS, Saeian K, Verber MD, et al. Inhibitory control test is a simple method to diagnose minimal hepatic encephalopathy and predict development of overt hepatic encephalopathy. Am J Gastroenterol 2007;102(4):754–60.
49. Bajaj JS, Hafeezullah M, Franco J, et al. Inhibitory control test for the diagnosis of minimal hepatic encephalopathy. Gastroenterology 2008;135(5):1591–600. e1591.
50. Bajaj JS, Hafeezullah M, Zadvornova Y, et al. The effect of fatigue on driving skills in patients with hepatic encephalopathy. Am J Gastroenterol 2009;104(4): 898–905.

51. Rovira A, Alonso J, Cordoba J. MR imaging findings in hepatic encephalopathy. AJNR Am J Neuroradiol 2008;29(9):1612–21.
52. Poveda MJ, Bernabeu A, Concepcion L, et al. Brain edema dynamics in patients with overt hepatic encephalopathy a magnetic resonance imaging study. Neuroimage 2010;52(2):481–7.
53. Van der Rijt CC, Schalm SW, De Groot GH, et al. Objective measurement of hepatic encephalopathy by means of automated EEG analysis. Electroencephalogr Clin Neurophysiol 1984;57(5):423–6.
54. Weissenborn K, Scholz M, Hinrichs H, et al. Neurophysiological assessment of early hepatic encephalopathy. Electroencephalogr Clin Neurophysiol 1990; 75(4):289–95.
55. Montagnese S, Amodio P, Morgan MY. Methods for diagnosing hepatic encephalopathy in patients with cirrhosis: a multidimensional approach. Metab Brain Dis 2004;19(3–4):281–312.
56. Montagnese S, Jackson C, Morgan MY. Spatio-temporal decomposition of the electroencephalogram in patients with cirrhosis. J Hepatol 2007;46(3):447–58.
57. Bajaj JS. Review article: the modern management of hepatic encephalopathy. Aliment Pharmacol Ther 2010;31(5):537–47.
58. Hwang S, Lee SG, Park JI, et al. Continuous peritransplant assessment of consciousness using bispectral index monitoring for patients with fulminant hepatic failure undergoing urgent liver transplantation. Clin Transplant 2010; 24(1):91–7.
59. Dahaba AA, Worm HC, Zhu SM, et al. Sensitivity and specificity of bispectral index for classification of overt hepatic encephalopathy: a multicentre, observer blinded, validation study. Gut 2008;57(1):77–83.
60. Patterson TL, Harvey P. Real-world functioning and self-evaluation of functioning: brain structure, mood state, functional skills, and mortality. Am J Geriatr Psychiatry 2008;16(8):617–20.
61. Grigsby J, Kaye K, Baxter J, et al. Executive cognitive abilities and functional status among community-dwelling older persons in the San Luis Valley Health and Aging Study. J Am Geriatr Soc 1998;46(5):590–6.

Assessment of Minimal Hepatic Encephalopathy (with Emphasis on Computerized Psychometric Tests)

Matthew R. Kappus, MD, Jasmohan S. Bajaj, MD, Msc*

KEYWORDS

- Minimal hepatic encephalopathy • Diagnosis
- Computerized testing • Cognition • Inhibitory control test
- Cognitive drug research system • Critical flicker frequency

Hepatic encephalopathy (HE) consists of a spectrum of neuropsychiatric abnormalities seen in patients with advanced liver disease, and is diagnosed after the exclusion of other known brain disease.[1] Whereas overt hepatic encephalopathy (OHE) is often diagnosed clinically, minimal hepatic encephalopathy (MHE) is more difficult to diagnose and more often requires the use of specialized testing to do so. MHE is regarded as a preclinical stage of OHE,[2] and results in a spectrum of cognitive deficits known as SONIC (Spectrum of Neurocognitive Impairment in Cirrhosis),[3] particularly in the domains of attention, vigilance, response inhibition, and executive function.[4–7] This sector of the continuum is being better recognized as having significant impact on quality of life in patients with cirrhosis. It is thought that approximately 60% to 80% of tested patients with cirrhosis have evidence of cognitive impairment or MHE.[8] In addition to the burden on quality of life, patients with evidence of MHE have increased risk for progression to OHE, and pose a potential danger to themselves or the community in the operation of heavy equipment and a motor vehicle.[4] Not only does this clinical condition affect the individual and those individuals in their immediate vicinity, there is also resource demand on society at large as costs increase to care for patients who ultimately have a high risk of developing OHE.[2]

Disclosures: Dr Kappus has nothing to disclose. Dr Bajaj has received grant funding from Salix Pharmaceuticals and Ocera Therapeutics.
Division of Gastroenterology, Hepatology and Nutrition, McGuire VA Medical Center, Virginia Commonwealth University, 1201 Broad Rock Boulevard, Richmond, VA 23249, USA
* Corresponding author.
E-mail address: jsbajaj@vcu.edu

Clin Liver Dis 16 (2012) 43–55
doi:10.1016/j.cld.2011.12.002
1089-3261/12/$ – see front matter © 2012 Elsevier Inc. All rights reserved.

The first challenge to treating these patients is identification and diagnosis. Diagnosis of MHE remains difficult, and most patients with cirrhosis are not routinely tested.[9–11] The reasoning for this lies in the time, psychological expertise, and financial burden of copyright constraints of administering the psychometric tests recommended by the Working Group on Hepatic Encephalopathy.[1] The Working Group on Hepatic Encephalopathy divided the diagnosis of HE into 3 categories: A (acute liver failure), B (portosystemic bypass without liver disease), and C (cirrhosis).[1] This article reviews the literature pertaining to group C, cirrhosis, from 2001 to 2011. These groups are clinically divided into episodic or persistent HE depending on their chronicity and minimal HE. Also included is any key information outside this date range.

SPECIFIC TESTING FOR CIRRHOSIS AND NORMAL MENTAL STATUS

As previously discussed, the Working Group on Hepatic Encephalopathy updated the classification of HE, which differentiates the stages of MHE and OHE.[1] The differentiation between a normal patient and one with subtle neurocognitive changes is a difficult task, and can only be defined by the presence of specific changes on psychometric testing and attention deficits.[5] Attention deficits play a role in a patient's ability to orient and perform executive functions, and impair learning and working memory.[12] These neurocognitive changes also involve defects in visuomotor coordination and response inhibition, both of which are important when operating a motor vehicle safely.[13–16] The investigation of these problems can only be done by the application of neuropsychometric or neurophysiologic testing, and the current repertoire includes the use of both traditional pen-paper and computerized testing (**Fig. 1, Table 1**).

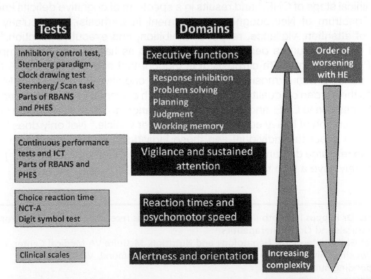

Fig. 1. Progression of severity of disease and appropriate testing strategies for each stage. (*Reprinted from* Bajaj JS, Wade JB, Sanyal AJ. Spectrum of neurocognitive impairment in cirrhosis: implications for the assessment of hepatic encephalopathy. Hepatology 2009;50: 2014–21; with permission.)

PAPER AND PENCIL PSYCHOMETRIC TESTS FOR MHE
Psychometric Hepatic Encephalopathy Score

Several batteries for the diagnosis of HE have been studied, and center around detection of deficits in attention and processing speed.[17] These tests identify impairments in visuospatial function, attention, response time, and inhibition, and are sensitive to the changes associated with MHE. The Psychometric Hepatic Encephalopathy Score (PHES) was specifically designed to detect changes associated with MHE, and comprises 5 different tests: the number connection test A (NCT-A), the number connection test B (NCT-B), the digit symbol test (DST), the line-tracing test (LTT), and the serial dotting test (SDT). Each of the different examinations tests for deficits in different areas: NCT-A and NCT-B evaluate concentration, mental tracking, and visuomotor speed. NCT-B does this with greater complexity. The DST evaluates psychomotor and visuomotor speed, whereas the LTT examines visuomotor and visuospatial skills with attention given to speed and accuracy. Lastly, the SDT is a test of psychomotor speed. Each test is scored on a scale of 1 to -3, according to standard deviation. Score ranges are between $+6$ and -18, with the determining value for pathologic condition at -4 points. This score has a sensitivity of 96% and specificity of 100%, with validation in several different countries, such as Germany, Italy, and Spain.[5,18,19] This test has not yet been validated in the United States.[1] If the PHES is unable to be completed, the Working Group on Hepatic Encephalopathy has recommended a combination of 2 of the following 4 tests: NCT-A, NCT-B, DST, or block design test (BDT). The recommendation is that impairment in at least 2 of these tests 2 standard deviations beyond age-matched controls of the same education indicates dysfunction.[1] The disadvantages of the PHES is that it is time consuming, not widely available in the United States, a poor test in memory, and often difficult to interpret. As an advantage, it is the current gold standard endorsed by the Working Party at the 1998 World Congress of Gastroenterology.

Rather than performing the PHES, Riggio and colleagues[20] performed a logistical regression analysis by first incorporating the scores of the 5 tests included in the PHES, and subsequently eliminating stepwise those variables that could be removed without impairing regression; this was called the Simplified Psychometric Hepatic Encephalopathy Score (SPHES). The logistic analysis in this study showed that a model containing only the DST, the SDT, and the LTT was similar to that containing the whole set of tests.[20] This factor is important in simplifying a test that is already highly regarded for being able to diagnose MHE. However, SPHES includes the LTT, which is the test that requires the longest to score, and there is controversy as to how to interpret its 2 outcomes: time and errors. The use of the SPHES decreased the time required for MHE screening but, because the NCT-A and B only require a maximum of 3 minutes, the practical utility of this reduction is not certain.

Repeatable Battery for Assessment of Neurologic Status

Another paper and pencil test recently recommended for use in the diagnosis of MHE is the Repeatable Battery for the Assessment of Neuropsychological Status (RBANS). The International Society for the Study of Hepatic Encephalopathy and Nitrogen Metabolism has recommended that this test, originally designed to diagnose neurocognitive disorders such as dementia, traumatic brain injury, stroke, multiple sclerosis, and bipolar disorder, be an alternative to PHES.[21] The RBANS has not been formally compared with the PHES, and has been the alternative in the United States. It has been used in several studies in the United States as an effective tool for screening for MHE[22,23]; however, it has not been formally compared with the PHES head to

Table 1
Characteristics of methods used to diagnose MHE

Test	Domains Tested	United States Norms	Copyright	Specialized Expertise (Psychology/ Neurology) Needed	Time for Administration Interpretation	Specific Comments
Paper-pencil psychometric tests						
NCT-A (number connection test A)	Psychomotor speed	+	No	No	30–120 s	Poor specificity
NCT-B (number connection test B)	Psychomotor speed, set shifting, and divided attention	–	Yes	Yes	1–3 min	More specific than NCT-A but is not pathognomonic for any disorder
BDT (block design test)	Visuospatial reasoning, praxis, and psychomotor speed	+	Yes	Yes	10–20 min	It can be used for dementia testing as well
DST (digit symbol test)	Psychomotor speed and attention	+	Yes	Yes	2 min	Tends to be very sensitive and is an early indicator
LTT (line-tracing test)	Psychomotor speed, and visuospatial	–	Yes	No	10 min	Outcomes are errors and time; tests the balance between speed and accuracy
SDT (serial dotting test)	Psychomotor speed	–	Yes	No	1–4 min	Only tests psychomotor speed
RBANS (Repeatable Battery for Assessment of Neuropsychological Status)	Verbal/visual/working memory, visuospatial, language, and psychomotor speed	+	Yes	Yes	35 min	Has been primarily studied in dementia and brain injury, current trials with HE are under way

Computerized Psychometric Tests						
ICT	Response inhibition, working memory, vigilance, and attention	Limited norms	Yes	No	15 min	Need highly functional patients, familiarity with computers may be needed
CDR	Attention and episodic and working memory	—	Yes	No	15–20 min	
Sternberg paradigm or Scan test	Working memory, vigilance, and attention	—	Yes	No	10–15 min	
Neurophysiologic Tests						
EEG MDF and spectral index	Generalized brain activity	Local norms	No	Yes	Different ranges	Can be performed in comatose patients
Visual evoked potentials	Interval between visual stimulus and activity	Local norms	No	Yes	Different ranges	Highly variable and poor overall results
Brainstem auditory evoked potentials	Response in the cortex after auditory click stimuli	Local norms	No	Yes	Different ranges	Inconsistent response with HE testing/prognostication
P300 cognitive evoked potentials	An infrequent stimulus embedded in irrelevant stimuli is studied	Local norms	No	Yes	Different ranges	Good diagnostic potential but requires patient cooperation
CFF	Visual discrimination and general arousal	—	No	No	10 min	Needs highly functional patients

NCT-A, NCT-B, DST, LTT, and SDT are parts of the Psychometric Hepatic Encephalopathy Score (PHES). Expense for each test depends on local availability, the need for copyrighted test materials, and computers. Up-front costs may be minimal if these tests are used often.

Abbreviations: BDT, block design test; CDR, cognitive disease research; CFF, critical flicker fusion frequency; DST, digit symbol test; EEG, electroencephalogram; HE, hepatic encephalopathy; ICT, inhibitory control test; LTT, line-tracing test; MDF, mean dominant frequency; NCT-A/-B, number connection tests A, B; RBANS, Repeatable Battery for Assessment of Neuropsychological Status; SDT, serial dotting test.

Reprinted from Bajaj JS, Wade JB, Sanyal AJ. Spectrum of neurocognitive impairment in cirrhosis: implications for the assessment of hepatic encephalopathy. Hepatology 2009;50:2014–21; with permission.

head. The test itself is divided into cortical and subcortical domains, and patients with HE perform worse on the subcortical components.[21] Although both of these examinations are able to provide information in detecting the diagnosis of MHE, in the United States both require a psychologist to order, administer, and interpret. Therefore, a movement toward computerized testing has the potential to expedite both administration and interpretation of MHE and HE.

COMPUTERIZED PSYCHOMETRIC TESTS

Paper and pencil tests rely heavily on the motor function and involve multiple cognitive functions for their completion. Efforts to overcome this issue have applied the use of reaction time,[24–26] which may take advantage of computerized testing and simple button pushing on the part of the patient. Reduced peripheral motor skills have the potential for complicating the interpretation of cognitive function, which is the goal of these tests. Computerized testing would simplify motor response, and may give information about other aspects of cognitive ability such as reaction time. The following are available computerized tests for the diagnosis of HE.

Choice Tests and Sternberg Paradigm

Amodio and colleagues[27] used a series of 3 computerized tests known as the Scan, Choice 1, and Choice 2 tests in a group of 94 patients with cirrhosis. They then followed the patients for overall survival and compared these tests with the NCT-A. The Scan test is based on the Sternberg paradigm in which the aim is to recognize whether there is at least a common number is pairs that are presented on the computer screen (most often "1" and "3"). The mean reaction times and percentage of errors are recorded. The test was performed by displaying a series of 72 random, sorted pairs of numbers for 3 seconds on the screen. The Choice tests 1 and 2 differed on difficulty of the task. Choice 1 measured the mean reaction times and the percentage of errors when pressing the same digit (between 1 and 4) on the keyboard, which was displayed for 3 seconds. Choice 2 measured the reaction times as well as the percentage errors when a reverse sequence of what was displayed on the screen was displayed. These tests used a weighted reaction time (Rt) as their outcomes. The team found that the NCT-A, Choice 2, and Scan tests were related to the severity of liver disease, which was not affected by disease etiology. Of note, the team found that overall survival was associated with alteration in the Scan test (hazard ratio 2.4) and Choice 2 (Hazard ratio 2.8) along with the Child Class. This test, however, needs to be validated in other populations.

Inhibitory Control Test

As mentioned earlier, the computerized psychometric tests have been developed over the last 6 years, and have the opportunity to change the face of how MHE is diagnosed. The inhibitory control test (ICT) is a computerized test of attention and response inhibition that has been used to characterize attention-deficit disorder, schizophrenia, and traumatic brain injury.[6,28–30] ICT measures response to lures and targets, and reaction times to provide an objective measurement of separate but complementary aspects of impairment in MHE. The lure response is an act of commission, signifying a defect in response inhibition.[31] Response inhibition is an essential aspect of executive function, which allows a subject to inhibit an incorrect response.[7,32] Impairment of response inhibition is responsible for potentiating wrong decisions in psychometric testing and in everyday life, and the ICT has been able to also quantify these errors in MHE.[4,33] The ICT also measures target detection rate, and errors in not detecting targets are considered errors of omission. These errors are considered primary errors of attention. Errors of omission are commonly associated with diminished processing speed and impairment of visuomotor function.[28] Both outcomes provide information about separate but complementary aspects of impairment in MHE.

The test consists in the presentation of several letters at 500-millisecond intervals, with the letters X and Y interspersed. The subject is instructed to respond to every X and Y during the initial part of the training program, thus establishing the prepotent response. In the latter part of the training run, the subject is instructed only to respond when X and Y are alternating (targets) and to desist from responding when X and Y are not alternating (lures) (**Fig. 2**). Typically, 6 test runs are completed by the patient, lasting 2 minutes, with a total of 40 lures, 212 targets, and 1728 random letters in between. At the test's conclusion, the lure and target response rates and the lure and target reaction times are automatically calculated. Good psychometric testing will depict lower lure response, higher target response, and shorter lure and target reaction times.

The ICT has been used in 2 centers in the Unites States, and results are also available from 2 Italian centers. The results from the United States were based on the analysis of more than 200 patients with varying degrees of cirrhosis and HE compared with healthy, age-matched and education-matched controls. The initial testing was performed using the NCT-A, DST, and BDT as gold standards. Using just the ICT lures in the United States population, there was good sensitivity and specificity for the diagnosis of MHE. There was a significantly lower target response and higher lure and target reaction times in MHE patients compared with others, but they did not add to the differentiation between the groups. The same group found that ICT lures were equivalent to the standard battery in predicting development of overt HE. The ICT has also been externally validated when applied to those patients who have received the transvenous intrahepatic portosystemic shunt (TIPS) procedure and those treated with probiotic therapy and rifaximin.[4,34] There is correlation with worsened response

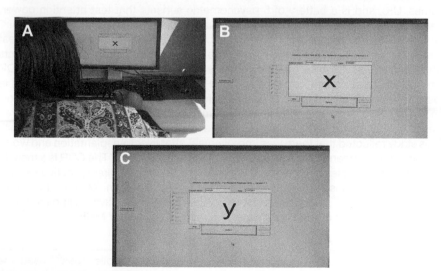

Fig. 2. The inhibitory control test (ICT). (*A*) Picture of a subject taking the ICT on a computer screen. (*B*) The appearance of the letter X on the computer screen during the ICT. (*C*) The appearance of the letter Y on the computer screen during the ICT.

to lures in patients' status post TIPS procedure, and improved lure response in patients treated with probiotic therapy.[4] Both of these observations are important, as one can see that change in disease status changes test findings.

ICT is a computerized instrument with automated analysis. Therefore, interobserver/ intraobserver reliability is not important. Studies conducted thus far have shown a high correlation of ICT lures and targets between administrations, indicating good test-retest reliability.[4,33] Studies have shown that the ICT is correlated with driving impairment on a simulator as well as with actual traffic accidents on a retrospective and prospective analysis.[14,16] Both of these findings suggest that ICT may be useful not only in the clinical setting for diagnostic purposes, but also in the trial setting. The experience of the Italian investigators was different with ICT because their population was significantly more advanced clinically, and had a lower educational background and exposure to computers.[35] These investigators concluded that a weighted lure (lures divided by the square of target accuracy) was a better differentiator of MHE in their patient population. Like Bajaj and colleagues,[4] they also did not find any difference in ICT outcomes between alcoholic and nonalcoholic etiology. The utility of ICT may be attributable to the difficulty of resource availability for the other psychometric tests, such as PHES, in the United States. A modified version of the ICT is available as a free download at www.hecme.tv, and may be administered on a personal computer. A further advantage is that ICT administration can be taught to an untrained, MA-level provider in approximately 30 minutes, as opposed to the necessary use of a trained psychologist for the administration of more traditional tests. The resources of both time and personnel have tremendous implications for the cost and logistical plausibility of being able to obtain the diagnosis of MHE in the clinical setting, and to properly address the needs of the patient. In addition, because ICT involves recognizing specific letters, it can potentially be administered to non–English-speaking subjects with minimal modifications.

Cognitive Drug Research Computerized Assessment System

This system was developed by Cognitive Drug Research Ltd (CDR, Goring-on-Thames, UK), and is a battery of 5 psychometric subsets that test attention power, attention continuity, speed of memory, and quality of episodic and working memory.[36] With more than 50 parallel forms of each task, the CDR system has been used to test cognitive function in clinical trials,[37] as well as neuropsychiatric conditions in patients with cirrhosis.[38] In 2008, a comparison was done between the utility of the CDR computerized assessment battery and the PHES for measuring cognitive function in those patients with cirrhosis being evaluated for liver transplantation or elective insertion or follow-up of a TIPS.[36] The test is administered on a computer and requires a yes/no response, requiring no prior computer experience from patients. The results of this study reflected that there was improvement after liver transplantation and worsening after the nitrogen challenge, status post TIPS procedure.[36] The CDR is simple to administer, requiring less than 30 minutes; however, it does require a practice session in advance. This test is currently available in the United Kingdom. With reliable correlation with the PHES,[36] good test-retest reliability, and high sensitivity in impaired populations,[39] the CDR is a good candidate as a diagnostic tool for MHE.

ImPACT Assessment System

In a study published only in abstract form, Tsushima and colleagues[40] used the ImPACT (Immediate Post-concussion Assessment and Cognitive Testing), a brief, validated, Web-based, computerized module that is validated for concussion. It is a 6-module neuropsychological test battery resulting in 4 composite scores (Verbal

Memory [VrbM], Visual Memory [VisM], Visual Motor Speed [VMS], and Reaction Time [RT]) with a normative group. These investigators compared 90 patients with cirrhosis with 131 controls, and found that the ImPACT scores significantly correlated with those of a standard battery (NCT-A/B and DST). They also found an association between ImPACT scores and quality of life. However, published studies on ImPACT in MHE and validation in other centers are awaited before this test can be used freely.

ELECTROPHYSIOLOGIC ASSESSMENT
Electroencephalogram

Neurophysiologic testing may be offered for the diagnosis of HE with the assistance of a neurologist and specialized staff, as well as dedicated equipment. This testing provides objective information on metabolic function, electrolyte homeostasis, and the effect of drugs and toxins on the brain. This examination is free of educational and cultural confounders when compared with psychometric examinations, as previously mentioned. In 1957, Parsons-Smith and colleagues[41] first noted slowing of the electroencephalography (EEG) rhythms in 40% of patients with cirrhosis, as well as EEG changes and HE severity. Further advances in EEG and the use of spectral EEG analysis have allowed for more accurate measurements of abnormalities present in cirrhosis.[18,42,43] The use of the Short Epoch Dominant Activity Clustering Algorithm (SEDECA) has subsequently provided a means for spatially mapping these deficits.[44] Recently, much work has been done to better define the neurophysiologic profile of patients with cirrhosis, specifically with regard to the examination of the usefulness of the EEG in routine workup of patients with cirrhosis. It has been shown that there seem to be associations between severity of liver disease and HE and alterations in EEG.[45]

Studies have shown that patients with cirrhosis have a reduced mean dominant frequency, higher theta relative power, and lower beta relative power in the parietal regions when compared with controls. The power of the spectral bands was similar in patients and controls over the frontal EEG regions.[45] As the degree of cirrhosis increased, there was associated slowing of the EEG rhythms, particularly in the parietal regions, and patients with a history of overt HE had an increase in negative changes in EEG readings in comparison with those without overt HE. At the conclusion of this study, prognosis and mortality were evaluated in light of changes in the EEG. The EEG may provide valuable prognostic information about both survival and the risk of overt HE.[45]

With the proper equipment and supervising personnel, the EEG may provide additional information with regard to neurophysiology during cirrhosis and HE. One thing to consider is that EEG examines only cortical activity, and therefore lacks the subcortical activity examination done with psychometric batteries such as the portosystemic encephalopathy syndrome test.[18] Psychometric batteries have been shown to often be more sensitive than neurophysiologic testing; however, there may be promise in measuring evoked potentials with EEG. Evoked potentials are the measurements of the time between a given stimulus (visual, somatosensory, and auditory) and the brain's ability to sense it. These potentials are divided into cortical and subcortical components, which would be helpful in narrowing the gap between psychometric and physiologic testing.[18] Visual evoked potentials have been found to only be useful in detecting early HE stages[46]; however, auditory responses to stimuli, measured as the auditory P300, have good diagnostic potential and can be used when available. The visual P300 is not recommended because of its inconsistent results.[47]

CRITICAL FLICKER FREQUENCY

Because of the lack of availability of the aforementioned neuropsychometric and physiologic tests due to a myriad of issues (copyrights, equipment, and proper personnel to administer them), recent studies have been performed examining tests that might be applied in the clinical setting by clinicians other than psychologists and/or neurologists. The critical flicker frequency (CFF) measures function at the level of the cortex, and has direct correlation with psychometric tests.[48] This test applies the theory that the pathogenesis of HE comprises low-grade astrocyte swelling,[49] disrupting neuronal communication. This same process occurs in glial cells of the retina.[50,51] The underlying thought is that retinal gliopathy could serve as a marker of cerebral gliopathy occurring in HE, and has been investigated in patients with low-grade HE.

The test is conducted by introducing a flickering light to the patient with a portable device, and the patient indicates the minimum frequency at which the light is still perceived as flickering and not fused. The frequency of the flickering is increased from 25 Hz onwards, and the patient determines the fusion-frequency threshold. The reverse is also undertaken, whereby the frequency of the light flickering is started at 60 Hz and the patient determines when the fused flickering light switches to being nonfused. The range of 38 to 39 Hz can differentiate between HE and no HE, but is less sensitive in differentiating MHE from HE. Results have been robust in both Spain and India.[52] This test is simple to administer, and may be deployed without the supervision or interpretation of a psychologist or neurologist. The test can be performed in a short period of time and, aside from the equipment, is not costly to perform. The CFF test, however, has not been validated for use in the United States population.

SUMMARY

The diagnosis of MHE remains an important challenge that needs to be faced, to evaluate the epidemic of patients with cirrhosis with this condition. These subtle changes in cognition require specialized testing, therefore expertise in this field is necessary to evaluate MHE in the clinical arena. There are several psychometric and neurophysiologic tests available to diagnose MHE, but there is currently no consensus regarding their use. The challenge for the future is to develop methods that properly evaluate cognitive function in HE as a continuum, as part of the SONIC,[3] to expedite diagnosis for determining outcome and administering proper treatment in a timely fashion.

REFERENCES

1. Ferenci P, Lockwood A, Mullen K, et al. Hepatic encephalopathy—definition, nomenclature, diagnosis, and quantification: final report of the working party at the 11th World Congresses of Gastroenterology, Vienna, 1998. Hepatology 2002; 35:716–21.
2. Poordad FF. Review article: the burden of hepatic encephalopathy. Aliment Pharmacol Ther 2007;25(Suppl 1):3–9.
3. Bajaj JS, Wade JB, Sanyal AJ. Spectrum of neurocognitive impairment in cirrhosis: implications for the assessment of hepatic encephalopathy. Hepatology 2009;50:2014–21.
4. Bajaj JS, Hafeezullah M, Franco J, et al. Inhibitory control test for the diagnosis of minimal hepatic encephalopathy. Gastroenterology 2008;135:1591–1600.e1.
5. Weissenborn K, Ennon JC, Schomerus H, et al. Neuropsychological characterization of hepatic encephalopathy. J Hepatol 2001;34:768–73.

6. Ford JM, Gray M, Whitfield SL, et al. Acquiring and inhibiting prepotent responses in schizophrenia: event-related brain potentials and functional magnetic resonance imaging. Arch Gen Psychiatry 2004;61:119–29.

7. Schiff S, Vallesi A, Mapelli D, et al. Impairment of response inhibition precedes motor alteration in the early stage of liver cirrhosis: a behavioral and electrophysiological study. Metab Brain Dis 2005;20:381–92.

8. Ortiz M, Jacas C, Cordoba J. Minimal hepatic encephalopathy: diagnosis, clinical significance and recommendations. J Hepatol 2005;42(Suppl):S45–53.

9. Saxena N, Bhatia M, Joshi YK, et al. Electrophysiological and neuropsychological tests for the diagnosis of subclinical hepatic encephalopathy and prediction of overt encephalopathy. Liver 2002;22:190–7.

10. Vergara-Gomez M, Flavia-Olivella M, Gil-Prades, et al. Diagnosis and treatment of hepatic encephalopathy in Spain: results of a survey of hepatologists. Gastroenterol Hepatol 2006;29:1–6.

11. Bajaj JS, Etemadian A, Hafeezullah M, et al. Testing for minimal hepatic encephalopathy in the United States: an AASLD survey. Hepatology 2007;45:833–4.

12. Amodio P, Schiff S, Del Piccolo F, et al. Attention dysfunction in cirrhotic patients: an inquiry on the role of executive control, attention orienting and focusing. Metab Brain Dis 2005;20:115–27.

13. Bajaj JS. Minimal hepatic encephalopathy matters in daily life. World J Gastroenterol 2008;14:3609–15.

14. Bajaj JS, Hafeezullah M, Hoffmann RG, et al. Minimal hepatic encephalopathy: a vehicle for accidents and traffic violations. Am J Gastroenterol 2007;102: 1903–9.

15. Bajaj JS, Hafeezullah M, Hoffmann RG, et al. Navigation skill impairment: another dimension of the driving difficulties in minimal hepatic encephalopathy. Hepatology 2008;47:596–604.

16. Bajaj JS, Saeian K, Schubert CM, et al. Minimal hepatic encephalopathy is associated with motor vehicle crashes: the reality beyond the driving test. Hepatology 2009;50:1175–83.

17. Ortiz M, Córdoba J, Doval E, et al. Development of a clinical hepatic encephalopathy staging scale. Aliment Pharmacol Ther 2007;26(6):859–67.

18. Amodio P, Campagna F, Olianas S, et al. Detection of minimal hepatic encephalopathy: normalization and optimization of the Psychometric Hepatic Encephalopathy Score. A neuropsychological and quantified EEG study. J Hepatol 2008;49:346–53.

19. Romero-Gomez M, Córdoba J, Jover R, et al. Value of the critical flicker frequency in patients with minimal hepatic encephalopathy. Hepatology 2007;45:879–85.

20. Riggio O, Ridola L, Pasquale C, et al. A simplified psychometric evaluation for the diagnosis of minimal hepatic encephalopathy. Clin Gastroenterol Hepatol 2011;9: 613–616.e1.

21. Sotil EU, Gottstein J, Ayala E, et al. Impact of preoperative overt hepatic encephalopathy on neurocognitive function after liver transplantation. Liver Transpl 2009; 15:184–92.

22. Sorrell JH, Zolnikov BJ, Sharma A, et al. Cognitive impairment in people diagnosed with end-stage liver disease evaluated for liver transplantation. Psychiatry Clin Neurosci 2006;60:174–81.

23. Meyer T, Eshelman A, Abouljoud M. Neuropsychological changes in a large sample of liver transplant candidates. Transplant Proc 2006;38:3559–60.

24. Douglass A, Al Mardini H, Record C. Amino acid challenge in patients with cirrhosis: a model for the assessment of treatments for hepatic encephalopathy. J Hepatol 2001;34:658–64.

25. Oppong KN, Al-Mardini H, Thick M, et al. Oral glutamine challenge in cirrhotics pre- and post-liver transplantation: a psychometric and analyzed EEG study. Hepatology 1997;26:870–6.
26. Rees CJ, Oppong K, Al Mardini H, et al. Effect of L-ornithine-L-aspartate on patients with and without TIPS undergoing glutamine challenge: a double blind, placebo controlled trial. Gut 2000;47:571–4.
27. Amodio P, Del Piccolo F, Marchetti P, et al. Clinical features and survival of cirrhotic patients with subclinical cognitive alterations detected by the number connection test and computerized psychometric tests. Hepatology 1999;29:1662–7.
28. Garavan H, Ross TJ, Stein EA. Right hemispheric dominance of inhibitory control: an event-related functional MRI study. Proc Natl Acad Sci U S A 1999;96:8301–6.
29. Konrad K, Gauggel S, Manz A, et al. Inhibitory control in children with traumatic brain injury (TBI) and children with attention deficit/hyperactivity disorder (ADHD). Brain Inj 2000;14:859–75.
30. Pliszka SR, Liotti M, Woldorff MG. Inhibitory control in children with attention-deficit/hyperactivity disorder: event-related potentials identify the processing component and timing of an impaired right-frontal response-inhibition mechanism. Biol Psychiatry 2000;48:238–46.
31. Ballard JC. Assessing attention: comparison of response-inhibition and traditional continuous performance tests. J Clin Exp Neuropsychol 2001;23:331–50.
32. Walker AJ, Shores EA, Trollor JN, et al. Neuropsychological functioning of adults with attention deficit hyperactivity disorder. J Clin Exp Neuropsychol 2000;22:115–24.
33. Bajaj JS, Saeian K, Verber MD, et al. Inhibitory control test is a simple method to diagnose minimal hepatic encephalopathy and predict development of overt hepatic encephalopathy. Am J Gastroenterol 2007;102:754–60.
34. Bajaj JS, Heuman DM, Wade JB, et al. Rifaximin improves driving simulator performance in a randomized trial of patients with minimal hepatic encephalopathy. Gastroenterology 2011;140:478–487.e1.
35. Amodio P, Ridola L, Schiff S, et al. Improving the inhibitory control task to detect minimal hepatic encephalopathy. Gastroenterology 2010;139:510–8, 518.e1–2.
36. Mardini H, Saxby BK, Record CO. Computerized psychometric testing in minimal encephalopathy and modulation by nitrogen challenge and liver transplant. Gastroenterology 2008;135:1582–90.
37. McKeith I, Del Ser T, Spano P, et al. Efficacy of rivastigmine in dementia with Lewy bodies: a randomised, double-blind, placebo-controlled international study. Lancet 2000;356:2031–6.
38. Forton DM, Thomas HC, Murphy CA, et al. Hepatitis C and cognitive impairment in a cohort of patients with mild liver disease. Hepatology 2002;35:433–9.
39. Wesnes KA, McKeith IG, Ferrara R, et al. Effects of rivastigmine on cognitive function in dementia with Lewy bodies: a randomised placebo-controlled international study using the cognitive drug research computerised assessment system. Dement Geriatr Cogn Disord 2002;13:183–92.
40. Tsushima M, Tsushima W, Tsushima V, et al. A case control study of ImPACT: a brief and effective web-based neuropsychological assessment battery to diagnose minimal hepatic encephalopathy (MHE) [Abstract]. J Hepatol 2010; 52(Suppl 1):S87.
41. Parsons-Smith BG, Summerskill WH, Dawson AM, et al. The electroencephalograph in liver disease. Lancet 1957;273:867–71.
42. Quero JC, Hartmann IJ, Meulstee J, et al. The diagnosis of subclinical hepatic encephalopathy in patients with cirrhosis using neuropsychological tests and automated electroencephalogram analysis. Hepatology 1990;24:556–60.

43. Van der Rijt CC, Schalm SW, De Groot GH, et al. Objective measurement of hepatic encephalopathy by means of automated EEG analysis. Electroencephalogr Clin Neurophysiol 1984;57:423–6.
44. Montagnese S, Jackson C, Morgan MY. Spatio-temporal decomposition of the electroencephalogram in patients with cirrhosis. J Hepatol 2007;46:447–58.
45. Marchetti P, D'Avanzo C, Orsato R, et al. Electroencephalography alterations in patients with cirrhosis. Gastroenterology 2011;141:1680–9.
46. Amodio P, Del Piccolo F, Pettenò E, et al. Prevalence and prognostic value of quantified electroencephalogram (EEG) alterations in cirrhotic patients. J Hepatol 2001;35:37–45.
47. Montagnese S, Amodio P, Morgan MY. Methods for diagnosing hepatic encephalopathy in patients with cirrhosis: a multidimensional approach. Metab Brain Dis 2004;19:281–312.
48. Kircheis G, Wettstein M, Timmermann L, et al. Critical flicker frequency for quantification of low-grade hepatic encephalopathy. Hepatology 2002;35:357–66.
49. Haussinger D, Kircheis G, Fischer R, et al. Hepatic encephalopathy in chronic liver disease: a clinical manifestation of astrocyte swelling and low-grade cerebral edema? J Hepatol 2000;32:1035–8.
50. Eckstein AK, Reichenbach A, Jacobi P, et al. Hepatic retinopathia. Changes in retinal function. Vision Res 1997;37:1699–706.
51. Reichenbach A, Fuchs U, Kasper M, et al. Hepatic retinopathy: morphological features of retinal glial (Muller) cells accompanying hepatic failure. Acta Neuropathol 1995;90:273–81.
52. Sharma P, Sharma BC, Puri V, et al. Critical flicker frequency: diagnostic tool for minimal hepatic encephalopathy. J Hepatol 2007;47:67–73.

Brain Imaging and Hepatic Encephalopathy

Mark J.W. McPhail, PhD, MRCP*, Neeral R. Patel, BSc,
Simon D. Taylor-Robinson, MD, FRCP

KEYWORDS

- Hepatic encephalopathy • Brain imaging
- Magnetic resonance imaging
- Magnetic resonance spectroscopy • Computed tomography
- Single-photon emission computed tomography
- Positron emission tomography

Hepatic encephalopathy (HE) is a neuropsychiatric disturbance affecting patients with acute liver failure (ALF), cirrhosis, or non–cirrhotic portosystemic bypass.[1] The clinical spectrum of HE extends from mild cognitive impairment to coma and death.[2] Most cases involve patients with minimal HE (MHE), which has been associated with an impaired ability to drive automobiles safely, reduced health-related quality of life, and an increased risk of hospitalization caused by overt HE.[3–5]

The disease process is multifactorial, with hyperammonemia, gut-derived toxins, short and medium chain fatty acids, cerebral manganese deposition, and relative deficiencies in circulating amino acids with consequent neurotransmitter imbalance commonly implicated. There is consensus that ammonia is central to the pathogenesis.[6] Varying degrees of cerebral edema may result from the uptake of excess ammonia into astrocytes, with subsequent conversion to glutamine (Gln), which acts as a cerebral osmolyte, mitochondrial toxin, and instigator of neurotransmitter instability.[7–11]

Currently, the diagnosis of HE lacks standardization, particularly in MHE, which requires neuropsychiatric testing to detect cognitive impairment. Psychometric test results can be dependent on the patients' age, educational status, emotional affect, and linguistic abilities. Evaluation varies between countries, although in some forms of testing, considerable expertise and facilities to conduct an assessment are required.[12] This perceived diagnostic difficulty leads to underrecognition of this important clinical problem. Even when the presentation of HE is clinically overt, the grading and assessment of longitudinal change is subjective among clinicians and is also prone to disagreement or even misdiagnosis.[12]

MJWM is supported by a Fellowship from the Wellcome Trust, London, United Kingdom. SDT-R holds grants from the British Medical Research Council, the Wellcome Trust, the National Institute of Health Research of the United Kingdom (NIHR), and the Alan Morement Foundation (AMMF).
Liver and Antiviral Center, Department of Medicine, St Mary's Hospital Campus, Imperial College London, 10th Floor QEQM Wing, South Wharf Street, London W2 1NY, UK
* Corresponding author.
E-mail address: mark.mcphail@imperial.ac.uk

Clin Liver Dis 16 (2012) 57–72
doi:10.1016/j.cld.2011.12.001
1089-3261/12/$ – see front matter © 2012 Elsevier Inc. All rights reserved.

The cerebral insults secondary to hepatocellular failure or portosystemic shunting result in structural and functional abnormalities in the brain, which imaging may detect and quantify. Suitable modalities include magnetic resonance imaging (MRI), magnetic resonance spectroscopy (MRS), computed tomography (CT) in conjunction with positron emission tomography (PET), and single-photon emission computed tomography (SPECT) (**Box 1, Table 1**). These imaging techniques may allow the development of tools for the objective, reproducible, and noninvasive diagnosis and monitoring of HE. Although stand-alone CT is useful for determining gross structural lesions, such as cerebral edema in ALF or other pathologic conditions in patients with CLD, it is limited as a diagnostic and longitudinal research tool because of poor sensitivity and repeated exposure to ionizing radiation. MRI and PET/SPECT are, thus, the focus for this article, with particular focus on patients with HE secondary to cirrhosis whereby the most possibility for diagnostic doubt or pathophysiological disagreement exists.

MRI

MRI is currently the most frequently used imaging tool in HE research studies, and even standard clinical sequences can give information supporting a diagnosis of HE. A clinical set of sequences when requesting an MR brain study would usually consist of T_1- and T_2-weighted sequences as standard and a selection of more advanced T_2-weighted sequences, such as fluid attenuated inversion recovery (FLAIR) or diffusion-weighted imaging (DWI).

T_1-Weighted MRI

Bilateral and symmetric hyperintensity of the basal ganglia using T_1-weighted MRI sequences in patients with cirrhosis is an observation with some clinical utility (**Fig. 1**).[13–16] It has been postulated that excess circulating manganese is the cause of such hyperintensity, caused by reduced hepatobiliary excretion as a result of liver failure, and subsequent deposition in the basal ganglia where blood flux is high.[17,18] This theory has been corroborated by the correlation between blood and cerebrospinal fluid manganese levels with T_1-weighted hyperintensity and also the normalization of basal ganglia hyperintensity and blood levels of manganese after liver transplantation.[19–21]

However, the results of studies investigating the relationship between manganese-related pallidal hyperintensity and psychometric performance in HE are conflicting.[22,23] It is, therefore, unclear whether T_1-weighted hyperintensity represents a manifestation of HE or if it is an occurrence secondary to cirrhosis, cholestasis, or portosystemic shunting.[24,25] The preferential deposition of manganese in the basal ganglia has been suggested to be an explanation for the parkinsonianlike symptoms, which can arise as

---

Box 1
Clinical and research imaging techniques applied in the diagnosis of HE

- CT brain can demonstrate edema in ALF and assists in the differential diagnosis of neurologic impairment in cirrhosis.
- MR brain is not recommended routinely in ALF but can assist in the diagnosis of HE in cirrhosis whereby it is the preferred method of brain imaging.
- Quantification of cerebral metabolites or brain water is possible but not yet widely used diagnostically.
- PET/SPECT are powerful but expensive research tools.

Table 1
Approach to different imaging modalities in HE in clinical and investigative use

Imaging Technique	Availability	Findings in HE	Recommended in the Clinic
CT brain	Standard	Cerebral edema in ALF Rules out some common differential diagnoses	Yes
MRI brain			
T₁ weighted	Standard	Basal ganglia hypersensitivity (not HE specific) Cerebral edema in ALF Quantitative brain volume by research statistical methods	Yes (not in ALF)
T₂ weighted			
FLAIR	Standard	White matter lesions in cases of low-grade HE	Yes (not in ALF)
DWI	Standard	High ADC in CHE Low ADC in ALF	
Diffusion tensor imaging	Research	Increased mean diffusivity in corticospinal tracts	No
Magnetization transfer	Available in specialist centers	Low MTR in white matter	No
¹H MRS	Available in specialist centers	High Glx Low myo-inositol and choline in basal ganglia and frontal white matter	No
Functional MRI	Research	Deactivation of the default mode network, including the anterior cingulate	
Nuclear medicine			
PET	Research in HE	Reduced glucose uptake in the anterior cingulate	No
SPECT	Research in HE	Increased blood flow to the basal ganglia	No

Abbreviations: ADC, apparent diffusion coefficient; CHE, chronic HE; DWI, diffusion-weighted imaging; FLAIR, fluid attenuated inversion recovery; Glx, glutamine/glutamate; MTR, magnetic transfer ratio.

a result of HE.[26] So, although a useful adjunct, this lack of correlation with grades of HE makes a single T₁-weighted examination insufficient in MR brain in patients with cirrhosis.

T₂-Weighted MRI: Fast FLAIR Imaging

Fast FLAIR T₂-weighted imaging represents an MRI sequence that has been shown to be sensitive for the detection of diffuse high-intensity white matter lesions (WMLs).[27,28] WMLs may develop secondary to cerebrovascular small-vessel disease, which, neuropathologically, is a combination of reversible edema and irreversible neuronal

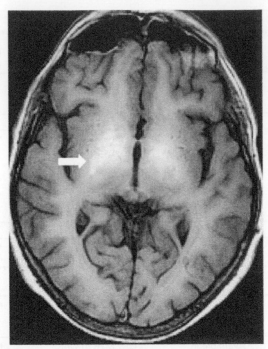

Fig. 1. T$_1$-weighted MRI of the brain of a patient with cirrhosis. The arrow demonstrates the area of pallidal hyperintensity. (*Reproduced from* Córdoba J, Sanpedro F, Alonso J, et al. 1H magnetic resonance in the study of hepatic encephalopathy in humans. Metab Brain Dis 2002;17(4):415; with permission from Springer Inc.)

damage.[29] Minguez and colleagues[30] noted WMLs were found to be reduced in volume and number after treatment with neomycin or branched-chain amino acids in conjunction with improved psychometric performance. To further investigate this observation, the same investigators compared WML volumes in patients with impaired cognition, before and after liver transplantation.[31] A significant reduction in WML volume was detected after liver transplantation (**Fig. 2**) as well as a strong negative correlation between fast FLAIR T$_2$-weighted lesion load and psychometric score. Rovira and colleagues[32] and Cordoba and colleagues[33] measured high-signal intensity along the corticospinal tract on fast FLAIR T$_2$-weighted images in patients with chronic liver disease with subsequent signal normalization after liver transplantation.

T$_2$-Weighted MRI: DWI

Diffusion-weighted MRI (DW-MRI) is a commonly available sequence often used in assessing neurovascular disease, which assesses changes in the motion of water molecules by defining the chemical interaction between water and cellular barriers.[34] The diffusivity of water molecules can be quantified by calculating the apparent diffusion coefficient (ADC) and can distinguish between vasogenic (interstitial) and cytotoxic edema.[35,36]

Several studies have consistently demonstrated a link between increased cerebral ADC (demonstrating interstitial edema) and patients with either MHE or overt HE, the degree of brain water diffusivity also correlating with the grade of HE.[36–39] DW-MRI studies have countered the traditional astrocytic swelling hypothesis, suggesting increased ADC values relate to purely extracellular water accumulation in low-grade

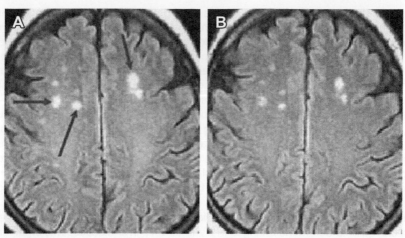

Fig. 2. (*A*) Baseline fast-FLAIR MRI image of a patient with hepatitis C before liver transplantation. Focal lesions can be visualized in the subcortical white matter (*arrows*). (*B*) Same MRI study 6 months after liver transplant in the same patient; there is a noticeable decrease in the size of focal white matter lesions. (*Reproduced from* Rovira A, Mínguez B, Aymerich FX, et al. Decreased white matter lesion volume and improved cognitive function after liver transplantation. Hepatology 2007;46(5):1485; with permission from John Wiley and Sons Inc.)

cerebral edema, secondary to chronic HE (CHE).[36,40–42] Theories that explain this phenomenon include hyperammonemia-induced increased blood-brain barrier permeability and reduced glial fibrillary acidic protein (GFAP) expression, a protein that regulates astrocytic permeability; reduced membranous GFAP in astrocytes has been previously linked to increased diffusivity in the extracellular space.[43–45] Discrepancies in studies whereby ADCs have been increased or decreased in clinically defined HE may be related to the onset of disease. Lower ADC values have been noted in patients with HE, secondary to ALF (and cytotoxic edema), whereas higher periventricular white matter and basal ganglia ADC in patients with CHE have been suggested to support a finding of interstitial edema.[46]

The detection of water diffusion has improved in recent years with the development of diffusion-tensor (DT) MRI, which is a technique that provides detailed information on brain tissue structure. Fractional anisotropy (whereby the fractional free or bound water component is estimated) maps can be assimilated to perform tractography, which is a method of determining the underlying brain anatomy and where edema is localized.[47] Kumar and colleagues[40] demonstrated increased mean diffusivity in the internal capsule and cortical gray and white matter of patients with HE, but differential patterns of correlation between mean diffusivity and fractional anisotropy in the corpus callosum suggested that interstitial edema was the primary HE correlate in this study of 14 patients with low-grade HE. Although DWI is often used in clinical scanners, and the authors would recommend using T_1-weighted and FLAIR/DWI T_2-weighted sequences, the statistical requirements of DT imaging (DTI) make it currently unsuitable for standard clinical use.

Volumetric MRI

Shah and colleagues[48] correlated quantitative T_1 mapping of cerebral water content in the putamen, globus pallidus, and occipital white matter with severity of HE. This measurement was one of the first direct and quantitative measurements of increased regional cerebral water content with more severe grades of HE, but the imaging technique is highly specialized. Cerebral edema that occurs as a result of ALF can be routinely viewed using MRI[49] but is often low grade and is, hence, undetectable by radiologists in CHE. The question arises about whether a simple measure of total brain volume (BV) would be useful. Recent developments in software packages for brain volumetry allow small (<1% total BV) changes in brain size in HE to be quantitated, allowing precise measurements of BV[50] on standard T_1-weighted MR sequences.[51–55] Single, time-point determination of BV is considerably less accurate than when BV change is determined longitudinally, owing to the ability to coregister (align) images using the theoretically unchanged skull surface, thus, allowing more robust determination of cerebrospinal fluid and gray and white matter densities.[50,56] Further structural information can be determined using voxel-based morphometry (VBM) whereby the regional contribution to BV change can be calculated; this has been applied in many neuropathologic scenarios.[57]

A pilot study conducted by Patel and colleagues[58] was the first to use coregistered MRI techniques to determine changes in BV in chronic liver disease. This small-scale investigation focused on 6 patients with MHE and 3 patients who had been diagnosed with overt HE. The investigators concluded that in patients treated with lactulose, BV decreased in association with improved psychometric performance.

In contrast, patients with HE often have risk factors for cerebral atrophy, such as age, alcohol abuse, and possibly cirrhosis itself, and these effects could also contribute to neuropsychologic impairment and apposite structural brain changes. Garcia-Martinez and colleagues[59] investigated cognitive function, cerebral MRS and BV after liver transplantation. After transplantation, BV was reduced in patients with prior HE, correlating with a worse neuropsychiatric score in this group. This study suggests that brain atrophy accrued before liver transplantation, but masked by low-grade edema, may also play a role in cognitive dysfunction after transplantation. Further evidence of the contribution of atrophy in patients with HE has recently emerged with the identification areas of atrophy throughout the cortex and white matter quantitated by VBM and correlating with the severity of encephalopathy.[60] A lack of corroborative MRS or more advanced water localization sequences could not add further mechanistic data to this interesting observation, which requires validation from other groups.

Magnetization Transfer Imaging

Magnetization transfer imaging (MTI) improves image contrast as a consequence of the magnetic properties of free and bound protons.[61] Free protons are present in water molecules, whereas bound protons are fixed to macromolecules, such as proteins, lipids, carbohydrates, and nucleic acids.[62] Magnetization transfer between bound and free protons reduces the signal intensity observed in the resultant MR image.[16,24] MTI also allows for the magnetic transfer ratio (MTR) to be quantified, which ultimately reflects brain parenchymal changes: a low MTR indicates neuronal damage as well as an increase in water content or membrane permeability.[16,63]

Lower MTRs have been demonstrated in patients with HE, including a cohort who developed MHE secondary to extrahepatic portal vein obstruction.[64–66] A study by Cordoba and colleagues[67] verified this by concluding MTR normalization after transplantation reflected the correction of low-grade cerebral edema in patients with MHE and that the basal ganglia and white matter are initial targets for water accumulation. A study by Miese and colleagues[39] that used both MTI and DW-MRI to investigate cerebral edema in HE found that both reduced MTR and raised ADC were correlated with HE grade in nonalcoholic patients. However, in patients continuing to drink alcohol to excess, no such correlation was established, suggesting chronic alcohol misuse may independently cause cerebral oxidative damage in this group, although as has been noted previously, the effect of atrophy on these measurements may be underestimated.[68]

Functional MRI

Functional MRI (fMRI) measures changes in deoxyhemoglobin concentration (a substance with paramagnetic properties relative to tissue) that occurs as a result of the increase in blood oxygenation during neuronal activity.[69] The subsequent blood-oxygen-level-dependent contrast highlights areas of activity in the brain.

fMRI has the benefit of being a noninvasive and safe investigatory tool in low-grade HE (because these patients can follow instructions in the scanner) that is particularly useful in longitudinal studies because no radioactive marker injections are required.[34] Zafiris and colleagues[70] demonstrated that MHE is associated with impaired coupling between visual judgment areas. A study conducted by Zhang and colleagues[71] compared brain fMRI data in 14 patients with cirrhosis and 14 healthy volunteers. An incongruous word-reading task and incongruous color-naming task (testing for attention and interference) highlighted various cerebral areas on fMRI: there was greater activation of the bilateral parietal and prefrontal cortices in the patients with cirrhosis.[72] In a separate study, Zhang and colleagues[73] concluded there was reduced functional connectivity in the right middle frontal gyrus and left posterior cingulate cortex, (part of the default-mode network). This highly interconnected, metabolically active, and well-described area of the brain is vital for the preservation of attention and is worthy of further study into whether this abnormal activation is related to hyper-ammonemia or low-grade cerebral edema.[74–76]

MRS

MRS has been used in HE investigations since the 1980s, although it has been more widely used in recent times as a consequence of improved sequence development and higher field strength to resolve metabolite signals. MRS also allows for the investigation of HE at the molecular level by studying cerebral tissue in vivo in whole-body clinical magnets (typically at 1.5–3.0 T).[77]

Various nuclei can be used to determine metabolite changes in HE, the most common clinically used being proton (^1H) and 31-phosphorus (^{31}P) MRS. ^1H MRS allows for the quantification of metabolites, such as choline (Cho), creatine (Cr), N-acetyl aspartate (NAA), Gln and glutamate (Glu), or the unresolved combination (Glx), as well as osmolytes, such as myo-inositol (mI) and taurine (Tau). ^{31}P MR spectra allow the definition of phosphomonoester (PME), inorganic phosphate (Pi), phosphodiester (PDE), phospho-creatine (PCr), γATP, αATP, and βATP resonances (or also more correctly termed nucle-oside triphosphate resonances [NTP] because they also contain contributions from cytosine triphosphate, guanosine triphosphate, and uridine triphosphate, in addition to the overwhelming proportion from adenosine triphosphate [ATP]).[78] These reso-nances provide information on cell membrane turnover with cell membrane precursors measured in the PME resonance and cell membrane degradation products measured in the PDE resonance, whereas information on high-energy phosphate metabolism and intracellular pH is available from the Pi, PCr, and NTP resonances.[79–81] Ammonia is not detected by MRS because of the rapid interchange with water.[82]

The characteristic spectral appearance of HE on in vivo ^1H MRS adds further evidence to the astrocyte swelling hypothesis demonstrated by a reduction in intracel-lular mI and Cho and a concurrent increase in Gln and Glu (**Fig. 3**).[78,83] Furthermore, these characteristic metabolic changes have been shown to correlate with psycho-metric performance.[22] This finding suggests that cells expel osmolytes, such as

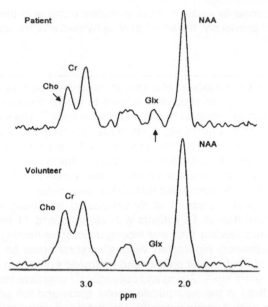

Fig. 3. ^{1}H MRS from the basal ganglia of a patient with CHE and a healthy volunteer, demonstrating decreased choline/creatine ratio and increased glutamate/glutamine resonance in the patient with CHE. (*Reproduced from* Taylor-Robinson SD, Sargentoni J, Marcus CD, et al. Regional variations in cerebral proton spectroscopy in patients with chronic hepatic encephalopathy. Metab Brain Dis 1994;9(4):347–59; with permission from Springer Inc.)

Tau, mI and Gln, in the face of an osmotic water load. In vivo ^{1}H MRS allows the degree of intracellular osmolyte homeostasis to be detected and monitored sequentially and to give an indirect indication of cell swelling in a noninvasive way. The technique is also open to following response to therapeutic intervention. Recent sequence development using 2-dimensional (2D) spectroscopy allows improved resolution of 1-dimensional ^{1}H MRS and resolution of Gln and Glu (**Fig. 4**).[84]

The interpretation of ^{31}P MRS is complex in vivo because many of the resonances are multi-component and are not easily separated into their constituents at clinically used magnetic field strengths. Overall, however, changes do seem to reflect alterations in bioenergetic pathways and glucose utilization (because sugar phosphates also contribute to both the PME and PDE resonances) as well as giving an indication of phospholipid membrane synthesis and degradation and of cell membrane fluidity.[78,85] Consensus on ^{31}P MRS studies has been hampered by small study sample sizes and inconsistencies in MRS protocols between centers.[34] Studies conducted by Taylor-Robinson and colleagues[78,85,86] have demonstrated reductions in the PME/βATP and PDE/βATP, which correlate with reduced Cho, as verified by parallel ^{1}H MRS on the same subjects. These changes were thought to represent reduced glucose utilization in HE because components of the glycolytic pathway contribute to the ^{31}P MRS spectrum in vivo. However, a change in membrane fluidity is equally possible. ^{1}H in vivo MRS is more likely to be developed for clinical use, but normal ranges and diagnostic thresholds for key metabolites are not yet agreed.

NUCLEAR MEDICINE: PET AND SPECT

PET involves the measurement of the concentration of positron-emitting radioisotopes from the body. Coregistered CT or MR tomographic imaging provides structural

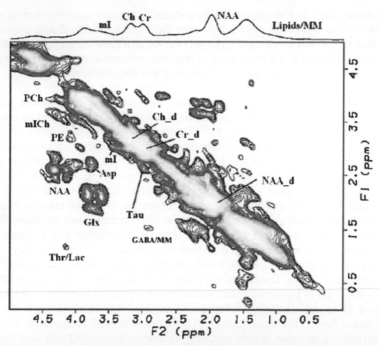

Fig. 4. The 2D-Correlation Spectroscopy spectrum from the occipital lobe of a 51-year-old patient with minimal HE. Asp, aspartate; GABA, gamma-aminobutyric acid; mICh, overlapping cross peaks of *myo*-inositol and choline; MM, macromolecules; PCh, phosphocholine; PE, phosphoethanolamine; ThrLac, overlapping cross peaks of threonine and lactate. (*Reproduced from* Singhal A, Nagarajan R, Hinkin CH, et al. Two-dimensional MR spectroscopy of minimal hepatic encephalopathy and neuropsychological correlates in vivo. J Magn Reson Imaging 2010;32(1):35; with permission from John Wiley and Sons Inc.)

information, whereas, depending on the radioligand used, functional data are available in the form of glucose and oxygen metabolism, blood flow, amino acid metabolism and rates of amino acid incorporation into proteins, acid-base balance, and membrane transport.[87] Positron-emitting radionuclides that are used in PET include ^{11}C, ^{18}F, ^{15}O, and [13]N.[88]

Lockwood and colleagues[89,90] have used ^{18}F-fluorodeoxyglucose (FDG) PET to investigate functional changes in CHE. They demonstrated a reduction in glucose metabolism in the anterior cingulate gyrus, which may reflect the attention deficit found in many patients with HE on neuropsychometric testing and in fMRI studies. Alterations in cerebral blood flow (CBF) have also been established using FDG PET and [15]O PET whereby poor neuropsychiatric performance correlated with reduced blood flow in all cortical areas; temporal lobe CBF was found to be most discriminatory between patients with HE and healthy volunteers.[89]

Brain imaging with ^{13}N-ammonia has been used to assess cerebral ammonia metabolism in (1) healthy subjects, (2) subjects with mild liver disease but with no evidence of cirrhosis, (3) subjects with cirrhosis with and without HE, and (4) subjects with malignant neoplasms with metastases in the liver.[91–95] However, the results of these studies are somewhat conflicting, particularly with respect to interpretation of blood-brain barrier (BBB) permeability in HE. This finding is probably because of the differences between research groups in the tracer kinetic modeling approach used to determine parameters of cerebral ammonia metabolism quantitatively. Different expert opinions exist over which conclusions should be drawn out of conflicting results in PET studies of ammonia metabolism and BBB permeability. Some proponents suggest that further studies, including larger numbers of patients and using standardized analysis techniques, are necessary to provide consensus and easy methodology to clarify the relationship between BBB permeability and ammonia toxicity.[96]

Changes in different neurotransmission systems have been demonstrated in patients with HE using radiotracer methods. Increased benzodiazepine receptor binding, decreased dopamine receptor binding, and decreased binding to serotonin transporters have been shown (**Fig. 5**).[97] These changes correspond to symptoms observed in HE (depression of neuropsychological function and extrapyramidal symptoms) and suggest possible targets for treatment.[98–100] Studies of neuronal activity have been used to shed light on the pathophysiology of HE, whereas imaging of a potentially crucial process in HE, neuroinflammation, using the radioligand C-11-PK11195 to detect peripheral benzodiazepine receptors, which are present on several cell types, including activated microglial cells, is gaining increased attention.[101–103]

Molecular imaging using SPECT requires a molecular marker that is labeled with a radionuclide, which results in the emission of gamma ray photons or high-energy x-ray photons.[104] Cerebral blood flow is most commonly assessed by using ^{99}Tc or ^{133}Xe radioactive tracers. Despite SPECT being more readily available and cheaper than PET, the latter is preferred in functional imaging studies because of its superior spatial and temporal resolution.[87] Previous studies have demonstrated increased cerebral blood flow in the basal ganglia in patients with MHE, suggesting increased ammonia delivery to these areas, resulting in astrocytic dysfunction and cognitive

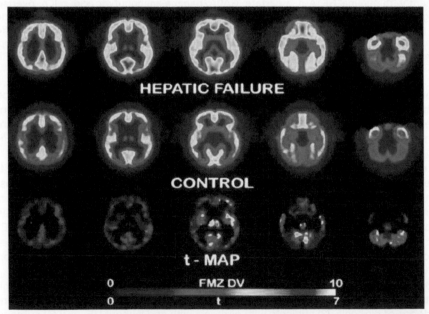

Fig. 5. Analyses of benzodiazepine binding in patients with hepatic failure (*top row*), control (*middle row*), and voxel-by-voxel comparison of between-group differences (*bottom row*). The greatest changes in distribution volume of flumazenil were seen in the cerebellum. (*Reproduced from* MacDonald GA, Frey KA, Agranoff BW, et al. Cerebral benzodiazepine receptor binding in vivo in patients with recurrent hepatic encephalopathy. Hepatology 1997;26(2):277; with permission from John Wiley and Sons Inc.)

alterations.[105,106] This finding is in agreement with a ^{1}H MRS study by Taylor-Robinson and colleagues[83] that demonstrated Glx concentration was highest in the basal ganglia. However, SPECT studies that have investigated HE have been thwarted by small study sizes, limiting the conclusions that can presently be drawn from the use of this functional imaging tool.

SUMMARY

In patients with liver disease and neurologic impairment, a CT scan or preferably MRI of the brain can rule out other diagnoses and provide some corroborative evidence of HE. More research-based modalities, such as MRT, DTI, MRS, PET, and SPECT, have provided valuable insight into the pathogenesis of HE but have not been transformed into widely available diagnostic tools. Before this transformation, there must be consensus regarding the uniformity of study protocols, imaging sequences, and analysis methodologies, both in MRI/MRS and in PET/SPECT, where promising functional data are emerging. In the future, a quantitative MR technique is most likely to give objective, reproducible, and longitudinal diagnostic information in this common but underrecognized complication of liver disease.

ACKNOWLEDGMENTS

All authors are grateful to the NIHR Biomedical Facility at Imperial College London for infrastructure support.

REFERENCES

1. Mullen KD. Review of the final report of the 1998 Working Party on definition, nomenclature and diagnosis of hepatic encephalopathy. Aliment Pharmacol Ther 2007;25:11–6.
2. Blei AT. Diagnosis and treatment of hepatic encephalopathy. Baillieres Best Pract Res Clin Gastroenterol 2000;14(6):959–74.
3. Bajaj JS, Saeian K, Schubert CM, et al. Minimal hepatic encephalopathy is associated with motor vehicle crashes: the reality beyond the driving test. Hepatology 2009;50(4):1175–83.
4. Bajaj JS, Hafeezullah M, Hoffmann RG, et al. Minimal hepatic encephalopathy: a vehicle for accidents and traffic violations. Am J Gastroenterol 2007;102(9):1903–9.
5. Prasad S, Dhiman RK, Duseja A, et al. Lactulose improves cognitive functions and health-related quality of life in patients with cirrhosis who have minimal hepatic encephalopathy. Hepatology 2007;45(3):549–59.
6. Lemberg A, Fernández MA. Hepatic encephalopathy, ammonia, glutamate, glutamine and oxidative stress. Ann Hepatol 2009;8(2):95–102.
7. Häussinger D, Kircheis G, Fischer R, et al. Hepatic encephalopathy in chronic liver disease: a clinical manifestation of astrocyte swelling and low-grade cerebral edema? J Hepatol 2000;32(6):1035–8.
8. Butterworth RF. Hepatic encephalopathy and brain edema in acute hepatic failure: does glutamate play a role? Hepatology 1997;25(4):1032–4.
9. Vaquero J, Chung C, Blei AT. Brain edema in acute liver failure. A window to the pathogenesis of hepatic encephalopathy. Ann Hepatol 2003;2(1):12–22.
10. Jones EA, Lavini C. Is cerebral edema a component of the syndrome of hepatic encephalopathy? Hepatology 2002;35(5):1270–3.
11. Häussinger D. Low grade cerebral edema and the pathogenesis of hepatic encephalopathy in cirrhosis. Hepatology 2006;43(6):1187–90.

12. Quero Guillen JC, Herrerías Gutiérrez JM. Diagnostic methods in hepatic encephalopathy. Clin Chim Acta 2006;365(1–2):1–8.

13. Zeneroli ML, Cioni G, Crisi G, et al. Globus pallidus alterations and brain atrophy in liver cirrhosis patients with encephalopathy: an MR imaging study. Magn Reson Imaging 1991;9(3):295–302.

14. Pujol A, Graus F, Peri J. Hyperintensity in the globus pallidus on T1-weighted and inversion-recovery MRI: a possible marker of advanced liver disease. Neurology 1991;41(9):1526–7.

15. Uchino A, Hasuo K, Matsumoto S, et al. Cerebral magnetic resonance imaging of liver cirrhosis patients. Clin Imaging 1994;18(2):123–30.

16. Córdoba J, Sanpedro F, Alonso J, et al. 1 H magnetic resonance in the study of hepatic encephalopathy in humans. Metab Brain Dis 2002;17(4):415–29.

17. Butterworth RF, Spahr L, Fontaine S, et al. Manganese toxicity, dopaminergic dysfunction and hepatic encephalopathy. Metab Brain Dis 1995;10(4):259–67.

18. Rose C, Butterworth RF, Zayed J, et al. Manganese deposition in basal ganglia structures results from both portal-systemic shunting and liver dysfunction. Gastroenterology 1999;117(3):640–4.

19. Spahr L, Butterworth RF, Fontaine S, et al. Increased blood manganese in cirrhotic patients: relationship to pallidal magnetic resonance signal hyperintensity and neurological symptoms. Hepatology 1996;24(5):1116–20.

20. Katsuragi T, Iseki E, Kosaka K, et al. Cerebrospinal fluid manganese concentrations in patients with symmetric pallidal hyperintensities on T1 weighted MRI. J Neurol Neurosurg Psychiatry 1999;66(4):551–2.

21. Pujol A, Pujol J, Graus F, et al. Hyperintense globus pallidus on T1-weighted MRI in cirrhotic patients is associated with severity of liver failure. Neurology 1993; 43(1):65–9.

22. Binesh N, Huda A, Thomas MA, et al. Hepatic encephalopathy: a neurochemical, neuroanatomical, and neuropsychological study. J Appl Clin Med Phys 2006; 7(1):86–96.

23. Weissenborn K, Ehrenheim C, Hori A, et al. Pallidal lesions in patients with liver cirrhosis: clinical and MRI evaluation. Metab Brain Dis 1995;10(3):219–31.

24. Taylor Robinson SD, Oatridge A, Hajnal JV, et al. MR imaging of the basal ganglia in chronic liver disease: correlation of T 1-weighted and magnetisation transfer contrast measurements with liver dysfunction and neuropsychiatric status. Metab Brain Dis 1995;10(2):175–88.

25. Forton DM, Patel N, Prince M, et al. Fatigue and primary biliary cirrhosis: association of globus pallidus magnetisation transfer ratio measurements with fatigue severity and blood manganese levels. Gut 2004;53(4):587–92.

26. Fabiani G, Rogacheski E, Wiederkehr JC, et al. Liver transplantation in a patient with rapid onset parkinsonism-dementia complex induced by manganism secondary to liver failure. Arq Neuropsiquiatr 2007;65(3A):685–8.

27. Bastianello S, Bozzao A, Paolillo A, et al. Fast spin-echo and fast fluid-attenuated inversion-recovery versus conventional spin-echo sequences for MR quantification of multiple sclerosis lesions. AJNR Am J Neuroradiol 1997; 18(4):699–704.

28. Rovaris M, Rocca MA, Yousry I, et al. Lesion load quantification on fast-FLAIR, rapid acquisition relaxation-enhanced, and gradient spin echo brain MRI scans from multiple sclerosis patients. Magn Reson Imaging 1999;17(8): 1105–10.

29. Englund E. Neuropathology of white matter lesions in vascular cognitive impairment. Cerebrovasc Dis 2000;13(2):11–5.

30. Minguez B, Rovira A, Alonso J, et al. Decrease in the volume of white matter lesions with improvement of hepatic encephalopathy. AJNR Am J Neuroradiol 2007;28(8):1499–500.
31. Rovira A, Mínguez B, Aymerich FX, et al. Decreased white matter lesion volume and improved cognitive function after liver transplantation. Hepatology 2007; 46(5):1485–90.
32. Rovira A, Córdoba J, Sanpedro F, et al. Normalization of T2 signal abnormalities in hemispheric white matter with liver transplant. Neurology 2002;59(3):335–41.
33. Córdoba J, Raguer N, Flavià M, et al. T2 hyperintensity along the cortico-spinal tract in cirrhosis relates to functional abnormalities. Hepatology 2003;38(4): 1026–33.
34. Grover VP, Dresner MA, Forton DM, et al. Current and future applications of magnetic resonance imaging and spectroscopy of the brain in hepatic encephalopathy. J Gastroenterol 2006;12(19):2969–78.
35. Schaefer PW, Grant PE, Gonzalez RG. Diffusion-weighted MR Imaging of the Brain. Radiology 2000;217(2):331–45.
36. Kale RA, Gupta RK, Saraswat VA, et al. Demonstration of interstitial cerebral edema with diffusion tensor MR imaging in type C hepatic encephalopathy. Hepatology 2006;43(4):698–706.
37. Sugimoto R, Iwasa M, Maeda M, et al. Value of the apparent diffusion coefficient for quantification of low-grade hepatic encephalopathy. Am J Gastroenterol 2008;103(6):1413–20.
38. Lodi R, Tonon C, Stracciari A, et al. Diffusion MRI shows increased water apparent diffusion coefficient in the brains of cirrhotics. Neurology 2004;62(5): 762–6.
39. Miese F, Kircheis G, Wittsack HJ, et al. 1H-MR spectroscopy, magnetization transfer, and diffusion-weighted imaging in alcoholic and nonalcoholic patients with cirrhosis with hepatic encephalopathy. AJNR Am J Neuroradiol 2006;27(5): 1019–26.
40. Kumar R, Gupta R, Elderkin-Thompson V, et al. Voxel-based diffusion tensor magnetic resonance imaging evaluation of low-grade hepatic encephalopathy. Journal of Magnetic Resonance Imaging 2008;27(5):1061–8.
41. Poveda MJ, Bernabeu A, Concepción L, et al. Brain edema dynamics in patients with overt hepatic encephalopathy: a magnetic resonance imaging study. Neuroimage 2010;52(2):481–7.
42. Mardini H, Smith FE, Record CO, et al. Magnetic resonance quantification of water and metabolites in the brain of cirrhotics following induced hyperammonaemia. J Hepatol 2011;54(6):1154–60.
43. Ziylan YZ, Uzm G, Bernard G, et al. Changes in the permeability of the blood-brain barrier in acute hyperammonemia. Effect of dexamethasone. Mol Chem Neuropathol 1993;20(3):203–18.
44. Sobel RA, DeArmond SJ, Forno LS, et al. Glial fibrillary acidic protein in hepatic encephalopathy an immunohistochemical study. J Neuropathol Exp Neurol 1981;40(6):625–32.
45. Chen KC, Nicholson C. Changes in brain cell shape create residual extracellular space volume and explain tortuosity behavior during osmotic challenge. Proc Natl Acad Sci U S A 2000;97(15):8306–11.
46. McKinney AM, Lohman BD, Sarikaya B, et al. Acute hepatic encephalopathy: diffusion-weighted and fluid-attenuated inversion recovery findings, and correlation with plasma ammonia level and clinical outcome. AJNR Am J Neuroradiol 2010;31(8):1471–9.

47. Nucifora PG, Verma R, Lee SK, et al. Diffusion-tensor MR imaging and tractography: exploring brain microstructure and connectivity. Radiology 2007;245(2): 367–84.
48. Shah NJ, Neeb H, Kircheis G, et al. Quantitative cerebral water content mapping in hepatic encephalopathy. Neuroimage 2008;41(3):706–17.
49. Fridman V, Galetta SL, Pruitt AA, et al. MRI findings associated with acute liver failure. Neurology 2009;72(24):2130–1.
50. Klauschen F, Goldman A, Barra V, et al. Evaluation of automated brain MR image segmentation and volumetry methods. Hum Brain Mapp 2009;30(4):1310–27.
51. Smith SM, Zhang Y, Jenkinson M, et al. Accurate, robust, and automated longitudinal and cross-sectional brain change analysis. Neuroimage 2002;17(1):479–89.
52. Smith SM, De Stefano N, Jenkinson M, et al. Normalized accurate measurement of longitudinal brain change. J Comput Assist Tomogr 2001;25(3):466–75.
53. Ashburner J, Friston KJ. Unified segmentation. Neuroimage 2005;26(3):839–51.
54. Dale AM, Fischl B, Sereno MI. Cortical surface-based analysis* I. Segmentation and surface reconstruction. Neuroimage 1999;9(2):179–94.
55. Fischl B, Sereno MI, Dale AM. Cortical surface-based analysis* II: Inflation, flattening, and a surface-based coordinate system. Neuroimage 1999;9(2):195–207.
56. Jenkinson M, Smith S. A global optimisation method for robust affine registration of brain images. Med Image Anal 2001;5(2):143–56.
57. Kakeda S, Korogi Y. The efficacy of a voxel-based morphometry on the analysis of imaging in schizophrenia, temporal lobe epilepsy, and Alzheimer's disease/mild cognitive impairment: a review. Neuroradiology 2010;52(8):711–21.
58. Patel N, White S, Dhanjal NS, et al. Changes in brain size in hepatic encephalopathy: a coregistered MRI study. Metab Brain Dis 2004;19(3):431–45.
59. GarciaMartinez R, Rovira A, Alonso J, et al. Hepatic encephalopathy is associated with posttransplant cognitive function and brain volume. Liver Transpl 2011;17(1):38–46.
60. Guevara M, Baccaro ME, Gómez-Ansón B, et al. Cerebral magnetic resonance imaging reveals marked abnormalities of brain tissue density in patients with cirrhosis without overt hepatic encephalopathy. J Hepatol 2011;55(3):564–73.
61. Pagani E, Bizzi A, Di Salle F, et al. Basic concepts of advanced MRI techniques. Neurol Sci 2008;29:290–5.
62. Wolff SD, Balaban RS. Magnetization transfer imaging: practical aspects and clinical applications. Radiology 1994;192(3):593–9.
63. Rovira A, Alonso J, Córdoba J. MR imaging findings in hepatic encephalopathy. AJNR Am J Neuroradiol 2008;29(9):1612–21.
64. Rovira A, Grive E, Pedraza S, et al. Spectroscopy of normal-appearing cerebral white matter in patients with liver cirrhosis. AJNR Am J Neuroradiol 2001;22(6):1137–42.
65. Miese FR, Wittsack HJ, Kircheis G, et al. Voxel-based analyses of magnetization transfer imaging of the brain in hepatic encephalopathy. World J Gastroenterol 2009;15(41):5157–64.
66. Goel A, Yadav S, Saraswat V, et al. Cerebral oedema in minimal hepatic encephalopathy due to extrahepatic portal venous obstruction. Liver Int 2010;30(8):1143–51.
67. Córdoba J, Alonso J, Rovira A, et al. The development of low-grade cerebral edema in cirrhosis is supported by the evolution of 1H-magnetic resonance abnormalities after liver transplantation. J Hepatol 2001;35(5):598–604.
68. Schweinsburg BC, Taylor MJ, Alhassoon OM, et al. Chemical pathology in brain white matter of recently detoxified alcoholics: a 1H magnetic resonance spectroscopy investigation of alcohol-associated frontal lobe injury. Alcohol Clin Exp Res 2001;25(6):924–34.

69. Howseman AM, Bowtell RW. Functional magnetic resonance imaging: imaging techniques and contrast mechanisms. Philos Trans R Soc Lond B Biol Sci 1999;354(1387):1179–94.
70. Zafiris O, Kircheis G, Rood HA, et al. Neural mechanism underlying impaired visual judgment in the dysmetabolic brain: an fMRI study. Neuroimage 2004; 22(2):541–52.
71. Zhang LJ, Yang G, Yin J, et al. Neural mechanism of cognitive control impairment in patients with hepatic cirrhosis: a functional magnetic resonance imaging study. Acta Radiol 2007;48(5):577–87.
72. MacLeod CM. Half a century of research on the Stroop effect: an integrative review. Psychol Bull 1991;109(2):163–203.
73. Zhang L, Qi R, Wu S, et al. Brain default-mode network abnormalities in hepatic encephalopathy: A resting-state functional MRI study. Hum Brain Mapp 2011. [Epub ahead of print]. DOI:10.1002/hbm.21295.
74. Power JD, Fair DA, Schlaggar BL, et al. The development of human functional brain networks. Neuron 2010;67(5):735.
75. Hafkemeijer A, van der Grond J, Rombouts SA. Imaging the default mode network in aging and dementia. Biochim Biophys Acta 2012;1822(3):431–41.
76. Broyd SJ, Demanuele C, Debener S, et al. Default-mode brain dysfunction in mental disorders: a systematic review. Neurosci Biobehav Rev 2009;33(3): 279–96.
77. McPhail MJ, Taylor-Robinson SD. The role of magnetic resonance imaging and spectroscopy in hepatic encephalopathy. Metab Brain Dis 2010;25(1):65–72.
78. Taylor-Robinson SD, Buckley C, Changani KK, et al. Cerebral proton and phosphorus-31 magnetic resonance spectroscopy in patients with subclinical hepatic encephalopathy. Liver 1999;19(5):389–98.
79. Patel N, Forton DM, Coutts GA, et al. Intracellular pH measurements of the whole head and the basal ganglia in chronic liver disease: a phosphorus-31 MR spectroscopy study. Metab Brain Dis 2000;15(3):223–40.
80. Hamilton G, Mathur R, Allsop JM, et al. Changes in brain intracellular pH and membrane phospholipids on oxygen therapy in hypoxic patients with chronic obstructive pulmonary disease. Metab Brain Dis 2003;18(1):95–109.
81. Hamilton G, Patel N, Forton DM, et al. Prior knowledge for time domain quantification of in vivo brain or liver 31P MR spectra. NMR Biomed 2003;16(3):168–76.
82. Cox IJ. Development and applications of in vivo clinical magnetic resonance spectroscopy. Prog Biophys Mol Biol 1996;65(1–2):45–81.
83. Taylor Robinson SD, Sargentoni J, Marcus CD, et al. Regional variations in cerebral proton spectroscopy in patients with chronic hepatic encephalopathy. Metab Brain Dis 1994;9(4):347–59.
84. Singhal A, Nagarajan R, Hinkin CH, et al. Two-dimensional MR spectroscopy of minimal hepatic encephalopathy and neuropsychological correlates in vivo. J Magn Reson Imaging 2010;32(1):35–43.
85. TaylorRobinson SD, Sargentoni J, Mallalieu RJ, et al. Cerebral phosphorus-31 magnetic resonance spectroscopy in patients with chronic hepatic encephalopathy. Hepatology 1994;20(5):1173–8.
86. Taylor Robinson SD, Sargentoni J, Oatridge A, et al. MR imaging and spectroscopy of the basal ganglia in chronic liver disease: correlation of T 1-weighted contrast measurements with abnormalities in proton and phosphorus-31 MR spectra. Metab Brain Dis 1996;11(3):249–68.
87. Stewart C, Reivich M, Lucey M, et al. Neuroimaging in hepatic encephalopathy. Clin Gastroenterol Hepatol 2005;3(3):197–207.

88. Miller PW, Long NJ, Vilar R, et al. Synthesis of 11C, 18F, 15O, and 13N radiolabels for positron emission tomography. Angew Chem Int Ed Engl 2008;47(47): 8998–9033.
89. Lockwood AH, Yap EW, Rhoades HM, et al. Altered cerebral blood flow and glucose metabolism in patients with liver disease and minimal encephalopathy. J Cereb Blood Flow Metab 1991;11(2):331–6.
90. Lockwood AH, Weissenborn K, Bokemeyer M, et al. Correlations between cerebral glucose metabolism and neuropsychological test performance in nonalcoholic cirrhotics. Metab Brain Dis 2002;17(1):29–40.
91. Ahl B, Weissenborn K, van den Hoff J, et al. Regional differences in cerebral blood flow and cerebral ammonia metabolism in patients with cirrhosis. Hepatology 2004;40(1):73–9.
92. Lockwood AH, McDonald JM, Reiman RE. The dynamics of ammonia metabolism in man. Effects of liver disease and hyperammonemia. J Clin Invest 1979; 63(3):449–60.
93. Lockwood AH, Bolomey L, Napoleon F. Blood-brain barrier to ammonia in humans. J Cereb Blood Flow Metab 1984;4(4):516–22.
94. Lockwood AH, Yap EW, Wong WH. Cerebral ammonia metabolism in patients with severe liver disease and minimal hepatic encephalopathy. J Cereb Blood Flow Metab 1991;11(2):337–41.
95. Keiding S, Sorensen M, Bender D, et al. Brain metabolism of 13N-ammonia during acute hepatic encephalopathy in cirrhosis measured by positron emission tomography. Hepatology 2006;43(1):42–50.
96. Berding G, Banati RB, Buchert R, et al. Radiotracer imaging studies in hepatic encephalopathy: ISHEN practice guidelines. Liver Int 2009;29(5):621–8.
97. Macdonald GA, Frey KA, Agranoff BW, et al. Cerebral benzodiazepine receptor binding in vivo in patients with recurrent hepatic encephalopathy. Hepatology 1997;26(2):277–82.
98. Jalan R, Turjanski N, Taylor-Robinson SD, et al. Increased availability of central benzodiazepine receptors in patients with chronic hepatic encephalopathy and alcohol related cirrhosis. Gut 2000;46(4):546–52.
99. Lozeva Thomas V. Serotonin brain circuits with a focus on hepatic encephalopathy. Metab Brain Dis 2004;19(3):413–20.
100. Weissenborn K, Berding G, Köstler H. Altered striatal dopamine D 2 receptor density and dopamine transport in a patient with hepatic encephalopathy. Metab Brain Dis 2000;15(3):173–8.
101. Cagnin A, Taylor-Robinson SD, Forton DM, et al. In vivo imaging of cerebral "peripheral benzodiazepine binding sites" in patients with hepatic encephalopathy. Gut 2006;55(4):547–53.
102. Desjardins P, Butterworth RF. The "peripheral-type" benzodiazepine (omega 3) receptor in hyperammonemic disorders. Neurochem Int 2002;41(2–3):109–14.
103. Iversen P, Hansen DA, Bender D, et al. Peripheral benzodiazepine receptors in the brain of cirrhosis patients with manifest hepatic encephalopathy. Eur J Nucl Med 2006;33(7):810–6.
104. Levin CS. Primer on molecular imaging technology. Eur J Nucl Med 2005;32:325–45.
105. O'Carroll RE, Hayes PC, Ebmeier KP, et al. Regional cerebral blood flow and cognitive function in patients with chronic liver disease. Lancet 1991;337(8752): 1250–3.
106. Catafau AM, Kulisevsky J, Bernà L, et al. Relationship between cerebral perfusion in frontal-limbic-basal ganglia circuits and neuropsychologic impairment in patients with subclinical hepatic encephalopathy. J Nucl Med 2000;41(3):405–10.

Management of Overt Hepatic Encephalopathy

Vandana Khungar, MD, MSc[a,b,*], Fred Poordad, MD[a,c]

KEYWORDS

- Hepatic encephalopathy • Liver disease • Cirrhosis
- Overt hepatic encephalopathy

Hepatic encephalopathy (HE) is a potentially reversible state of impaired cognitive function or altered consciousness in patients with liver disease or portosystemic shunting.[1] It represents a continuum of transient and reversible neurologic and psychiatric dysfunction, varying from subtly altered mental status to deep coma. It can be categorized into 3 types: type A, which occurs in acute liver failure; type B, which occurs in patients with bypass shunts; and type C, which occurs in patients with chronic liver disease.[2,3] Type C HE is of importance given the increasing burden of cirrhosis in the United States and the world. Approximately 5.5 million people in the United States have hepatic cirrhosis.[4] It is difficult to estimate the true incidence of HE, but the majority of patients with cirrhosis develop a degree of encephalopathy at some point during their disease. Overt HE (OHE) occurs in at least 30% to 45% of cirrhotic patients and 10% to 50% of patients with transjugular intrahepatic portosystemic shunt (TIPS).[5,6]

HE imposes a significant burden on patients, their families, and health care resources.[4,7] A recent 104-patient cross-sectional study in 2 transplant centers revealed that previous HE and cognitive dysfunction are associated with worse employment, financial status, and caregiver burden. Patients with previous HE had 87.5% unemployment versus 19% in those without previous HE ($P = .00001$). Patients with previous episodes of HE also had lower financial status and posed a higher caregiver burden than those who had not experienced HE.[8] Cognitive performance and Model for End-Stage Liver Disease (MELD) scores were significantly correlated with employment and caregiver burden.[8] Based on the Zarit short form, caregivers

---

[a] Department of Medicine, Cedars-Sinai Medical Center, 8635 West Third Street, Suite 1060, Los Angeles, CA 90048, USA
[b] Department of Medicine, David Geffen School of Medicine at UCLA, Los Angeles, CA, USA
[c] Department of Surgery, Cedars-Sinai Medical Center, 8635 West Third Street, Suite 1060, Los Angeles, CA 90048, USA
* Corresponding author. Department of Medicine, Cedars-Sinai Medical Center, 8635 West Third Street, Suite 1060, Los Angeles, CA 90048.
E-mail address: vandana.khungar@gmail.com

Clin Liver Dis 16 (2012) 73–89
doi:10.1016/j.cld.2011.12.007
1089-3261/12/$ – see front matter © 2012 Elsevier Inc. All rights reserved.

liver.theclinics.com

are at similar stress levels compared with caregivers of patients with Alzheimer disease (score 15 ± 10) and patients with advanced cancer (score 12 ± 8.5) but at lower stress levels compared with caregivers of patients with acute brain injury (score 21.7 ± 10.1).[9]

OHE is a particularly pressing problem. Episodes can occur without warning and often require inpatient hospitalization. In 2005, more than 50,000 patients required hospitalization for HE.[7] Increases in the frequency and severity of episodes of HE predict an increased risk of death.[10,11] Data presented at the 2010 annual meeting of the American Association for the Study of Liver Diseases and at the 2011 annual meeting of the European Association for the Study of the Liver (EASL) by Bajaj and colleagues[13] showed that deficits in working memory, psychomotor speed, attention, and response inhibition increase with the number and severity of episodes of OHE. It is possible that the metabolic derangements that produce OHE cause chronic neurologic injury that is not readily reversible.[12,13] For patients with severe HE who are hospitalized, 1-year and 3-year survival rates are less than 50% and less than 25%, respectively.[14]

DIAGNOSIS OF HE

OHE is diagnosed clinically, based on 2 types of symptoms: impaired mental status, as defined by the West Haven criteria (Conn score), and impaired neuromotor function.[4,15,16] The Working Party on Hepatic Encephalopathy recommends the Conn score for assessment of OHE in clinical trials.[3] More recently, the Hepatic Encephalopathy Scoring Algorithm has been used.[17] Examples of neuromotor impairment include hyperreflexia, rigidity, myoclonus, and asterixis.[16,18,19] OHE can be further subdivided into episodic or persistent and precipitated or spontaneously occurring.

THERAPY OF OVERT HE

The burden of OHE is great and the diagnosis simple. Clinicians must ensure that a patient has OHE, treat precipitating factors if necessary, triage the patient to an ICU versus floor bed, decide if intubation is necessary to protect the airway, and treat with appropriate pharmacotherapy. After an episode of OHE, prophylactic therapy with lactulose or rifaximin is recommended for an indefinite period of time or until liver transplantation. Currently available treatment strategies for OHE are presented in **Table 1**.

Clinical guidelines for OHE were published 10 years ago, and many physicians have developed comfort with older therapies.[20] As new therapies are discovered, practice patterns should change. The first step in treatment is identifying and treating precipitating causes, including but not limited to hypovolemia, gastrointestinal (GI) bleeding, infection, dehydration secondary to diuretic use, diarrhea, vomiting, hyponatremia, hypokalemia or hyperkalemia, alkalosis, surgery, renal failure, TIPS, constipation, benzodiazepine use, narcotic use, hypoxemia, hepatoma, and noncompliance with lactulose therapy.[21]

Therapy is generally focused on treating episodes after they occur. Many agents currently available reduce the nitrogenous load in the gut to reduce the accumulation of ammonia.[7,22] The 2 key therapies used to reduce circulating ammonia are nonabsorbable disaccharides and oral antibiotics. Both reduce intestinal production and absorption of ammonium ions (NH_4^+).[23] The standard of care has been nonabsorbable disaccharides (lactitol or lactulose), which decrease the absorption of ammonia through cathartic effects and by altering colonic pH.[20] Oral antibiotics have also proved useful in reducing ammonia-producing enteric bacteria.[20,24,25] The long-term use of some oral

Table 1
Therapeutic approaches for the treatment of overt hepatic encephalopathy

General supportive care	Fall precautions in disoriented patients Prevention of infections—changing IV lines, prevent aspiration pneumonia, isolation Monitor fluid status Maintain normoglycemia and electrolytes Correct alkalosis
Nutritional support	Energy intake of 35–40 kcal/kg bw/d and protein intake of 1.2–1.5 g/kg bw/d Consider addition of BCAAs, zinc; consider eliminating wheat and milk proteins
Treating precipitating events GI bleeding	Octreotide, IV PPI, endoscopic or angiographic therapy Blood transfusions, correction of coagulopathy NG lavage to remove blood from stomach
Infection	Antibiotic therapy
Sedating medications	Discontinue benzodiazepines, narcotics; consider flumazenil or naloxone
Electrolyte abnormalities	Discontinue diuretics; perform serial paracentesis if needed Correct hypokalemia or hyperkalemia, hyponatremia
Constipation	Provide laxatives and enemas
Renal failure	Discontinue diuretics Albumin administration Discontinue nephrotoxic medications
Ammonia excretion	Lactulose enemas
Ammonia production	Antibiotics—neomycin, paromomycin, metronidazole, vancomycin Minimally absorbed antibiotics—rifaximin Nonabsorbable disaccharides—lactulose, lactitol Probiotics—lactobacillus, bifidobacterium Ammonia scavengers—sodium benzoate, sodium phenylacetate, sodium phenylbutyrate AST-120, LOLA, LOPA, or OCR-002 α-Glucosidase inhibitor—acarbose Closure of spontaneous portal systemic shunt Liver transplantation Artificial liver support

Abbreviations: IV, intravenous; kg bw, kilograms body weight; NG, nasogastric; PPI, proton pump inhibitor.

antibiotics is not recommended because of nephrotoxicity, ototoxicity, and peripheral neuropathy. Rifaximin, a minimally absorbed oral antibiotic, has promise in treatment of OHE. Several randomized controlled trials (RCTs) have been performed on the therapies available and are summarized in **Table 2**.[33–36] A recent review recommended that treatment strategies should focus on management of precipitating factors, reduction of ammonia and other toxins, modulation of fecal flora, modulation of neurotransmission, correction of nutritional deficiencies, and reduction of inflammation.[2] Serial measurements of ammonia levels do not provide additional information beyond clinical assessment of the mental status and may not correlate well with clinical outcomes.[37,38]

Table 2
Selected randomized controlled trials of treatment of hepatic encephalopathy

Author	Design Description	Subject Characteristics	Results
Bass et al,[26] 2010, multinational	Double-blind, placebo-controlled trial to study rifaximin (550 mg bid) × 6 months vs placebo in secondary prophylaxis of HE	N = 299, 2 prior episodes of HE in current remission	Reduced risk of OHE in rifaximin group compared with placebo over 6-month period. HR 0.42 (95% CI, 0.28–0.64). NNT to prevent 1 episode of HE = 4; NNT to prevent 1 hospitalization = 9.
Riggio et al,[75] 2005, Italy	Double-blind, randomized trial to study lactitol (60 g/d) vs rifaximin (1200 mg/d) vs no treatment in prevention of post-TIPS HE	N = 75, cirrhotics who had undergone TIPS	1-Month HE incidence was similar in the 3 groups. Lactitol or rifaximin was not effective in the prophylaxis of HE during the 1st month after TIPS.
Malaguarnera et al,[74] 2011, Italy	Double-blind, placebo-controlled randomized trial to study ALC (2 g bid) vs placebo in severe HE	N = 61, severe HE (grade 3 on West Haven scale)	Statistically significant improvements in ALC group in memory, trail making test, controlled word association, Hooper Visual Organization Test, judgment of line orientation, digit cancellation time.
Sharma et al,[29] 2009, India	Open-label RCT of lactulose vs placebo for secondary prophylaxis of HE	N = 140, cirrhotics with previous episodes of HE	19.6% in the lactulose group vs 46.8% in the placebo group (P = .001) developed HE over a median follow-up of 14 months.
Kanematsu et al,[27] 1988, Japan	Randomized prospective study to evaluate BCAAs vs conventional amino acid solutions on postoperative HE	N = 56, cirrhotics undergoing surgery	3 in the BCAA group (10.3%) had HE; 3 in the control group (11.1%) had HE. There was no preventive effect noted with BCAAs.

Rolachon et al,[30] 1994, France	Randomized prospective trial to evaluate mannitol irrigation vs no irrigation	N = 40, cirrhotics with an upper GI bleed	In the mannitol group, there was significantly less HE (5% vs 30%) and lower length of stay (8.2 vs 13.6 days). Mortality was the same.
Uribe et al,[31] 1987, Mexico	Double-blind randomized trial to evaluate acidifying enemas vs tap water enemas to treat HE	N = 20, cirrhotics with at least West Haven grade 2 HE	In acidifying enema group, 86% of patients had a favorable response (similar for lactose and lactitol). The tap water group was stopped early due to significant failure.
Hassanein et al,[28] 2007, USA	Prospective, randomized, multicenter trial to study ECAD for severe HE, comparing ECAD and SMT vs SMT alone for 5 days	N = 70, cirrhotics with severe HE (grade 3/4)	Improvement proportion was higher in the ECAD group (mean 34% vs 18.9%) and was reached faster and more frequently than in SMT group. Survival not analyzed.
Kircheis et al,[32] 1997, Germany	Randomized, double-blind, placebo-controlled trial of IV LOLA for HE	N = 126, cirrhotics with chronic HE without known precipitants	OA showed significant improvement over placebo for ammonia concentrations, mental state gradation, and PSEI.
Stauch et al,[33] 1998, Germany	Randomized, double-blind, placebo-controlled trial of LOLA for chronic HE	N = 66, cirrhotics with HE	Number connection performance times, fasting and postprandial venous blood ammonia concentrations, mental state grade, and PSEI were significantly improved in the LOLA group.
Sushma et al,[34] 1992, India	Randomized double-blind trial to compare sodium benzoate to lactulose in the treatment of acute HE.	N = 74, cirrhotics with HE	Clinical, EEG, and psychometric test scores were similar in both groups as were side effects. The cost of lactulose was 30 times that of sodium benzoate.

(continued on next page)

Table 2
(continued)

Author	Design Description	Subject Characteristics	Results
Reding et al,[35] 1984, Belgium	Randomized, double-blind, placebo-controlled trial to assess zinc acetate (600 mg daily) for HE	N = 22, cirrhotics with chronic HE	Serum zinc restored to normal by day 8. HE assessed by trail test improved in zinc but not placebo group; increase in SUN in zinc group. The duration of improvement is unknown.
Riggio et al,[36] 1991, Italy	Randomized, double-blind, crossover, placebo-controlled trial to compare zinc sulfate (600 mg daily) with placebo for HE	N = 15, cirrhotics with chronic HE	Serum zinc was raised after oral zinc administration, but no modification in the Conn index was noted. No improvement was seen in HE.
Gentile et al,[55] 2005, Italy	Randomized, double-blind, crossover trial of acarbose (100 mg tid) vs placebo in cirrhotics with type 2 DM for HE	N = 107, cirrhotics with HE and type 2 DM	Acarbose significantly decreased ammonia blood levels and improved Reitan test score and intellectual function score compared with placebo.

Abbreviations: ALC, acetyl-L-carnitine; DM, diabetes mellitus; ECAD, extracorporeal albumin dialysis; HR, hazard ratio; PSEI, portal systemic encephalopathy index; SMT, standard medical therapy; SUN, serum urea nitrogen.

Management of Precipitating Factors

Breakthrough episodes of HE can be either precipitated by an identifiable event or occur spontaneously. Infection is the most commonly identified precipitant when there is one.[39,40] GI bleeding, both immediately after and for several days after the bleed, can precipitate HE; occult GI bleeding can lead to HE as well.[41] Dehydration resulting from aggressive diuresis with volume contraction alkalosis and electrolyte disturbances commonly causes HE in patients with ascites and edema. Patients who have had a TIPS procedure and whose medications are not appropriately adjusted after the procedure often develop HE. This type of HE responds well to fluid resuscitation and electrolyte repletion.[42] Albumin is particularly helpful in these patients whereas other colloids are not as useful.[43]

The risk of infection in hospitalized cirrhotic patients is approximately 5 times higher than in hospitalized noncirrhotic patients.[2] An aggressive investigation to find the infectious source must be conducted in patients with HE. Some physicians begin empiric antimicrobial therapy while body fluid analyses and cultures are performed, particularly when there are clinical features, such as fever, or laboratory changes, such as leukocytosis. A diagnostic paracentesis should be performed for any patient with ascites who presents with HE to rule out spontaneous bacterial peritonitis.

A generalized inflammatory state exists in cirrhotics, even without infection, with elevated levels of endotoxin, tumor necrosis factor (TNF)-α, inflammatory cytokines, and Toll-like receptors. The increase in inflammation may be due to bowel wall edema from portal hypertension or delayed transit time with subsequent translocation of bacteria or endotoxin into the systemic circulation. Antibiotics given to cirrhotics with HE may reduce this proinflammatory state. Other therapies with anti-inflammatory activity are pentoxifylline (anti–TNF-α) and the activated charcoal product AST-120 (Ocera Therapeutics). Pentoxifylline has not yet been studied as a therapy for HE. AST-120 may bind very small molecules in the gut, such as TNF-α, lipopolysaccharide, or endotoxin, and block their absorption. It is being evaluated in trials for the treatment of HE.[2]

Overzealous administration of lactulose can lead to hypokalemia from diarrhea, exacerbating HE. Repletion of electrolytes, in particular potassium, is key in treating HE. Potassium deficiency exacerbates hyperammonemia by up-regulating renal glutaminase and the production of ammonia.[2] Constipation is also thought to be a cause of HE, possibly by increasing the amount of time available for ammonia absorbed from the GI tract. Hyponatremia can precipitate HE but can also cause neurologic dysfunction, which may be difficult to differentiate clinically from HE. For patients with hypovolemia, treatment of hyponatremia is with intravenous saline whereas for those who are euvolemic or hypervolemic, water restriction or vasopressin antagonists are used.

An often-overlooked clinical scenario, particularly in the inpatient setting, is the use of sedating or hypnotic medications. Because cirrhotic patients have a higher incidence of anxiety, depression, pain disorders, and disrupted sleep-wake cycle, they are often given benzodiazepines or opiates, which can trigger HE.

Reduction of Ammonia by Nonabsorbable Disaccharides

Because ammonia is thought to be a key player in the development of HE, it is the target of the most widely used HE therapies, and decreased ammonia is used as a significant endpoint in many clinical trials assessing HE treatments. The degree of ammonia elevation has been associated with the stage of HE, although this is not as clear outside of research settings.[44,45] The correlation between degree of ammonia elevation and stage of HE is noted in particular in type A HE, where cerebral edema and death have been correlated with the degree of hyperammonemia.

Ammonia is derived from both intestinal flora and other sources, such as entero-cytes, in the small bowel and colon, which produce ammonia when they metabolize glutamine.[46] Ammonia may cause neurologic dysfunction by its effect on cerebral edema. Glutamine is produced within astrocytes in the brain from glutamate and ammonia. Glutamine in turn attracts water and causes swelling of astrocytes. Ammonia can then directly cause oxidative stress, up-regulating cytokine production, inflammatory responses, and impaired intracellular signaling. Ammonia can also be broken down by skeletal muscle, so in cirrhotic patients with a large degree of muscle wasting, it is more difficult to clear ammonia. For this reason, it is clinically appropriate to increase protein intake in cirrhotic patients to slow the rate of muscle loss. Testosterone levels can also be repleted when low.

The standard approach to reducing ammonia levels in type C HE has been to administer nonabsorbable disaccharides, such as lactulose (β-galactosidofructose) in the United States or lactitol (β-galactosidosorbitol) in Europe. They are thought to reduce ammonia levels by several mechanisms. They acidify and speed passage of the fecal stream through the colon and promote the growth of beneficial acid resistant, non–urease-producing bacteria. On entering the colon, lactulose is cleaved into mono-saccharides by the bacterial flora. Some bacteria, including *Lactobacilli* and *Bifidobac-teria*, can incorporate the monosaccharides into subsequent generations of bacteria, conferring a growth advantage. The unincorporated monosaccharides are also used as fuel for the bacteria. The fermentation generates lactic acid and hydrogen ions, acid-ifying the fecal stream, and causes protonation of the ammonia molecules (NH_3) into NH_4^+. The charged ammonium ions are difficult for colonocytes to absorb and remain trapped in the colonic lumen. The protonation also allows for movement of NH_3 from the bloodstream into the colonic lumen. Lactulose is also thought to transform fecal flora, with a reduction in urease-producing bacteria that are not given a growth advantage and an increase in the proteolytic species *Lactobacilli* and *Bifidobacteria*. The cathartic action of excessive amounts of lactulose can also promote the elimination of ammonia, although excessive diarrhea leads to dehydration, which can worsen HE.[47]

A Cochrane database systematic review of RCTs from 2004 did not show a signifi-cant survival benefit with the use of nonabsorbable disaccharides for the treatment of HE and showed that they were less effective than antibiotics for improving HE.[25,48] In a 125-patient open-label, single-site study, however, Sharma and colleagues showed that lactulose was more effective than placebo in the secondary prevention of OHE in the outpatient setting (19.6% vs 46.8% [$P = .001$]).[29]

Compliance with lactulose therapy is a concern because many of the side effects are difficult to tolerate. The most common side effects include an unpleasant sweet taste, bloating, flatulence, nausea, vomiting, and severe diarrhea, leading to dehydra-tion, hypokalemia, hypernatremia, and other electrolyte disturbances. Dehydration may worsen HE, lead to acute kidney injury, and precipitate hepatorenal syndrome. The dosages of lactulose in HE are 30 mL to 45 mL (20–30 g) 3 to 4 times daily. This amount should be titrated to produce 2 to 3 soft stools per day. Hourly doses should not be used to induce diarrhea as was common practice in years past, primarily due to the risk of exacerbating volume contraction and rapid shifts in electrolytes. A study of lactulose dosing at a large tertiary care center that specialized in liver disease showed great variability in dosing of lactulose. Inpatient orders for lactulose were retrospectively reviewed for 1 year, with a total of 5107 orders. Inappropriate dosing in the form of standing orders, single-dose orders, and as-needed orders was noted, suggesting that a standardized dosing order set may help prevent complications from inappropriate dosing.[20,49] Lactulose can be administered via enema when patients are too obtunded for oral intake. Enema administration can be difficult for nursing staff and has variable efficacy due to variation in dwell times and level of exposure to medication. It can, however, be an effective method for an obtunded patient if oral administration is not possible.

Reduction of Ammonia Levels by Ammonia Scavengers and Activated Charcoal

Intravenous sodium benzoate and sodium phenylacetate or the phenylacetate prodrug oral sodium phenylbutyrate can combine with glycine or glutamine to form water-soluble compounds excreted through the kidneys. These agents are not yet approved by the US Food and Drug Administration for this use; they depend on normal renal function for ammonia excretion, and the large therapeutic doses confer a significant sodium load, which can increase fluid retention. Newer ammonia scavengers and orally ingested activated charcoal are being studied.[2,50] Glycerol phenylbutyrate (HPN-100, Hyperion Therapeutics) is a new compound that is a prodrug of sodium phenylbutyrate with much lower therapeutic doses needed. It is being evaluated for type C HE and has done well in trials for urea cycle disorders.

Orally ingested activated charcoal is also being explored for the treatment of HE. AST-120 is a spherical carbon adsorbent being studied in patients with mild HE and cirrhotic patients with pruritus. The molecule adsorbs small molecules (ammonia, lipopolysaccharides, and cytokines), all of which may contribute to HE. A pilot study shows equal efficacy to lactulose and fewer adverse events (AEs).[43] In animal models, administration of AST-120 caused a reduction in ammonia and cerebral edema. The AST-120 Used to Treat Hepatic Encephalopathy (ASTUTE) trial, a human study of AST-120 in patients with mild type C HE, has recently been completed and results should be available soon.

Modulation of Fecal Flora with Oral Antibiotics, Prebiotics, Probiotics, and Acarbose

The gut microbiome plays a significant role in the pathogenesis of HE. The gut flora can be modified through antibiotics, probiotics, or prebiotics to alter the disease course. Prebiotics include lactulose and fermentable fibers and enhance the growth of bacterial strains that are potentially beneficial to the host and reduce more harmful flora, such as the urease-producing species.[51–53] Probiotics are not as useful in OHE but have been used with some success in minimal HE. The species that are most efficacious are *Lactobacilli* and *Bifidobacteria*. Probiotics may also reduce bacterial translocation and subsequent endotoxemia and ameliorate the hyperdynamic circulation.

Oral antibiotics have proved efficacy in treating OHE by reducing the number of ammonia-producing bacteria present in the gut. Neomycin has been used, but due to concerns over nephrotoxicity and ototoxicity of aminoglycosides, the use of this medication has been limited. This toxicity is considered cumulative, such that hearing loss, in particular, can occur slowly over time and is not reversible. The dose of neomycin used in most clinical trials was 3 g to 4 g daily, which is much higher than what most clinicians are accustomed to using in practice. Similarly, metronidazole is effective in treating HE, but concerns over resistance and peripheral neuropathy have limited its use.[54,55] Paramomycin and vancomycin have also been used, but there are concerns with their long-term use and bacterial resistance.

Acarbose, an α-glucosidase inhibitor, may be useful in the treatment of HE. By reducing glucose absorption from the gut, the survival of saccharolytic bacteria is favored over proteolytic bacteria, reducing the generation of ammonia. A randomized, double-blind, crossover trial of acarbose in diabetic patients with mild HE showed a decrease in ammonia levels and improvement in HE grade. These data are not yet compelling enough, however, to adopt the use of this compound.

Rifaximin

Rifaximin (Xifaxan, Salix Pharmaceuticals) has low systemic bioavailability, is concentrated in the GI tract, and has broad-spectrum in vitro activity against gram-positive and gram-negative aerobic and anaerobic enteric bacteria, with a low risk of bacterial resistance, making it a better choice for long-term treatment when compared to systemically absorbed antibiotics.[56–58] Its preferred site of action is the small bowel because it has enhanced solubility in bile. In the small bowel it lowers the bacterial load 100-fold to 1000-fold, but it is less effective in the colon. One possible mechanism of action of rifaximin in HE is the correction of small intestinal bacterial overgrowth. The benefit of antibiotics may result from the change in bowel flora, their anti-inflammatory effects or down-regulation of intestinal glutaminase activity. Rifaximin has been shown more efficacious than nonabsorbable disaccharides and equivalent efficacy to other antibiotics used in the treatment of acute HE. It has also been shown to improve health-related quality of life (HRQOL). In an assessment of 219 patients randomized to rifaximin or placebo, the majority of whom were on concomitant lactulose, Sanyal and colleagues[59,60] assessed quality of life. The Chronic Liver Disease Questionnaire was administered every 4 weeks and rifaximin significantly improved HRQOL in patients with cirrhosis and recurrent HE. A lower HRQOL may also predict recurrence of HE.[59,60] In the 299-patient randomized, double-blind, placebo-controlled, multinational phase 3 trial of rifaximin for remission from HE, Bass and colleagues[26] showed that rifaximin plus lactulose is superior to lactulose alone in the secondary prophylaxis of HE. The primary endpoint was time to first breakthrough episode of HE. The key secondary endpoint was time to first hospitalization involving HE. Rifaximin significantly reduced the risk of an episode of OHE compared with placebo over a 6-month period. The hazard ratio with rifaximin was 0.42 (95% CI, 0.28–0.64; $P<.001$). In 22.1% of the rifaximin group versus 45.9% of the placebo group, a breakthrough episode of HE occurred. Hospitalizations involving HE occurred in 13.6% of the rifaximin group and 22.6% of the placebo group, with a hazard ratio of 0.50 (95% CI, 0.29–0.87). In both groups, more than 90% of patients received concomitant lactulose therapy. The number needed to treat (NNT) to prevent one episode of HE is 4 and the NNT to prevent one hospitalization is 9. AEs and serious AEs (SAEs) were similar in the 2 groups.[26] Rifaximin, however, has not been studied in patients with MELD scores greater than 25, and 9% of patients in the trial had MELD scores greater than 19. There is a slightly higher systemic exposure of the drug in patients with Child-Pugh class C scores due to the biliary excretion of the drug. It is still a low exposure rate overall, and these patients can likely safely take the drug.

In an abstract presented at the 2011 EASL meeting annual meeting, Mullen and colleagues[61] demonstrated the long-term efficacy and survival in patients treated with rifaximin for the maintenance of remission from OHE. This study was an open-label maintenance extension of the phase 3 trial by Bass and colleagues.[26] The study included 322 patients: 70 from the RCT who continued rifaximin, 82 from the RCT who crossed over from the placebo arm, and 170 new patients. Average follow-up was 16 months, and some patients had up to 3 years of exposure. Across both the RCT and the current open-label study, mean duration of drug exposure among rifaximin-treated patients was 476 days, for a total of 510 person-exposure years. HE event rates (number of events per person years of exposure of the study drug) ranged from 0.24 to 0.40 in patients on rifaximin to 1.6 in those on placebo. In a pooled analysis, rifaximin was associated with a significant reduction in rates of hospitalization for any cause (0.45 events per person-exposure years with rifaximin vs 1.31 with placebo [P<.0001]) and rates of HE-related hospitalizations (0.21 vs 0.72 [P<.0001]). Rifaximin was associated with a lower AE rate compared with placebo (0.71 vs 2.8), lower drug-related AE rate (0.11 vs 0.74), lower SAE rate (0.48 vs 1.4), and lower rate of discontinuations due to AEs (0.25 vs 0.98). Rifaximin was not associated with increased mortality rates.[61]

The results of a case-control study of the long-term administration of rifaximin for patients with alcohol-related decompensated cirrhosis were presented at the 2011 EASL meeting. Vlachigiannakos and colleagues[62] showed that in a population of patients with alcohol-related cirrhosis who had been abstinent from alcohol for at least 6 months, during a follow-up period of 5 years, HE occurred in 31.5% in the rifaximin group versus 47.0% in the placebo group (P = .034).[62] More importantly, there were significantly fewer cases of portal hypertension–related events, such as variceal bleeds, spontaneous bacterial peritonitis, and hepatorenal syndrome. As a result, there was a significantly higher survival in patients treated with rifaximin. The probable mechanism of this change in portal hypertension–related events is due to a change in gut-derived bacterial cytokines, with resultant changes in hepatic venous gradient pressures. Another study by Leise and colleagues[63] revealed a 2-year survival advantage in more than 300 cirrhotic patients with moderate to severe HE treated with rifaximin, compared with more than 6500 patients on the US transplant wait list. These studies need to be validated but are intriguing and may help further clarify the true mechanism of action of rifaximin.

Modulation of Neurotransmission

HE is associated with up-regulation of γ-aminobutyric acid neuroinhibitory receptors and N-methyl-D-aspartic acid–glutamate excitatory receptors, resulting in confusion between inhibitory and excitatory signals. Trials have been completed with flumazenil, naloxone, bromocriptine, levodopa, and acetylcholinesterase (AChE) inhibitors, but none has had a large degree of success. In comatose patients with HE and benzodiazepine or opiate ingestion, a trial of flumazenil or naloxone is appropriate, with careful monitoring for seizures.[64,65] A pilot study of the AChE inhibitor rivastigmine in patients with moderate HE demonstrated an improvement in psychometric testing.[66]

Protein Restriction

Dietary protein restriction was once thought to reduce the nitrogenous load entering the gut, thereby reducing ammonia production and absorption and subsequent HE. It has now fallen out of favor because malnutrition as a result of protein restriction in cirrhotics has occurred. An RCT of protein-restricted diets and normal protein diets in cirrhotics with HE revealed no difference in the course of HE in the 2 groups. Higher protein breakdown was documented in the protein-restricted group.[67] Because poor nutritional status is a risk factor for mortality in cirrhotics, it is now recommended that cirrhotics with HE be given regular protein diets and medical therapy for the HE.[67,68]

An abstract presented at the 2011 EASL meeting from Balzola and colleagues[69] suggested that a wheat-free and milk-protein–free diet may be considered an adjunctive treatment of HE. Diets free of wheat or milk proteins have been shown to reduce blood concentrations of exogenous opioid peptides, which have a direct central morphine-like action. In this prospective study, patients with untreatable chronic HE awaiting liver transplantation were given a normoproteic diet that was free of wheat and milk proteins. After 4 weeks, 87% of patients had consistent clinical improvement.

After 3 months, complete resolution of HE was maintained in these patients. The significant improvements in global cognitive status with the diet were not associated with significant electroencephalographic (EEG) changes and rechallenge with a wheat and milk diet led to an HE event in 1 patient.[69]

Correction of Nutritional Deficiencies

Poor dietary absorption of fat-soluble vitamins; poor intake secondary to confusion, weakness, or ascites; and a baseline hypercatabolic state contribute to poor nutritional status in cirrhotics. Zinc serves as a cofactor in the urea cycle, and zinc deficiency, which is common in cirrhotics, may decrease efficiency of the urea cycle. A randomized open-label trial showed potential benefit in HE with zinc supplementation.[70]

Outside the United States, L-ornithine-L-aspartate (LOLA) is frequently used for HE. LOLA is believed to act by supplying substrates for the urea cycle and glutamine synthesis that are sometimes depleted in cirrhotics with protein malnutrition and amino acid deficiencies. A meta-analysis of 3 trials demonstrated significant benefit in patients with grade I-II HE.[71] L-ornithine phenylacetate (LOPA) or OCR-002 (Ocera Therapeutics) is similar to LOLA and is being developed and tested in HE. It may increase the amount of ornithine available in the urea cycle, enhancing the incorporation of ammonia into glutamine. Ammonia is scavenged by conjugating phenylacetate with glutamine to form phenylacetylglutamine, which is then excreted in the urine. A phase II trial will begin in 2011.[72]

The Fischer ratio is the balance between branched-chain amino acids (BCAAs) and aromatic amino acids. The ratio is usually 3:1 in a healthy population but is reversed in cirrhotics. The BCAAs—valine, leucine, and isoleucine—are necessary for protein production and for the prevention of catabolism. The aromatic amino acids are precursors of false neurotransmitters, octopamine and phenylethylamine, and have been implicated in HE because they can inhibit neurotransmission via competitive blockade of receptors. Supplementing diets with BCAAs may allow adequate protein intake and reduced catabolism and muscle breakdown and prevent synthesis of false neurotransmitters. A meta-analysis of BCAA supplementation showed improved rate of recovery from episodic HE but no survival advantage.[73]

One Italian center has reported its experience with L-carnitine or acetyl-L-carnitine. A double-blind, placebo-controlled RCT performed by this group demonstrated a significant improvement in EEG, cognitive deficits, and reduction of ammonia in the treated group for severe HE.[74]

Extracorporeal Liver Devices

The use of extracorporeal devices for liver dialysis is now being considered. The one system clinically available in the United States is the molecular adsorbent recirculating system (MARS, Gambro), otherwise known as albumin dialysis, and is indicated for acute liver toxicity. An RCT in the United States for patients with severe HE not responding to standard care showed quicker improvements in HE but no benefit in mortality.[28,75] Bioartificial machines with hepatocytes have been studied for HE but are not currently available in the United States.

Shunting

Some patients with persistent HE despite removal of precipitating factors and treatment with currently available medical therapies may have extensive portosystemic shunting. These shunts may be embolized via percutaneous catheterization, but this is not yet commonplace in the United States.

SUMMARY

Given the many targets of treatment and lack of a clear singular cause of OHE, there is no consensus on a single best treatment. The current management of OHE requires accurate and prompt diagnosis, elimination of precipitating factors, and administration of pharmacologic therapy tailored to a particular patient. In episodic or mild persistent HE, nonabsorbable disaccharides (lactulose and lactitol) remain the most widely prescribed medications, although this practice is changing toward using rifaximin as first-line therapy in many cases. Ammonia scavengers are useful for patients intolerant to lactulose and/or antibiotics or as adjunctive treatment in those already on lactulose and rifaximin. Nutritional supplementation with zinc or L-carnitine may be useful. AST-120, LOPA, acarbose, and rivastigmine are still under investigation. Patients with OHE should be considered for liver transplantation. Over the past several years, high-quality studies have been conducted on the various pharmacologic therapies for HE and as more data emerge, hopefully HE will become a much more easily treated complication of decompensated liver disease.

REFERENCES

1. Voight M, Conn H. Hepatic encephalopathy. In: Robson SC, Trey C, Kirsch RE, editors. Diagnosis and management of liver disease. London: Chapman & Hall; 1995. p. 140–7, Chapter 13.
2. Frederick RT. Current concepts in the pathophysiology and management of hepatic encephalopathy. Gastroenterol Hepatol 2011;7(4):222–33.
3. Ferenci P, Lockwood A, Mullen K, et al. Hepatic encephalopathy—definition, nomenclature, diagnosis and quantification: final report of the working party at the 11th World Congresses of Gastroenterology, Vienna 1998. Hepatology 2002;35:716–21.
4. Poordad FF. Review article: the burden of hepatic encephalopathy. Aliment Pharmacol Ther 2007;25(Suppl 1):3–9.
5. Romero-Gomez M, Boza F, Garcia-Valdecasas MS, et al. Subclinical hepatic encephalopathy predicts the development of overt hepatic encephalopathy. Am J Gastroenterol 2001;96:2718–23.
6. Boyer TD, Haskal ZJ. American Association for the Study of Liver Diseases. The role of transjugular intrahepatic portosystemic shunt in the management of portal hypertension. Hepatology 2005;41:386–400.
7. Leevy CB, Phillips JA. Hospitalizations during the use of rifaximin versus lactulose for the treatment of hepatic encephalopathy. Dig Dis Sci 2007;52:737–41.
8. Bajaj JS, Wade JB, Gibson DP, et al. The multi-dimensional burden of cirrhosis and hepatic encephalopathy on patients and caregivers. Am J Gastroenterol 2011;106:1646–53.
9. Higginson IJ, Gao W, Jackson D, et al. Short-form Zarit caregiver burden interviews were valid in advanced conditions. J Clin Epidemiol 2010;63:535–42.
10. Bustamante J, Rimola A, Ventura PJ, et al. Prognostic significance of hepatic encephalopathy in patients with cirrhosis. J Hepatol 1999;30:890–5.
11. Stewart CA, Malinchoc M, Kim WR, et al. Hepatic encephalopathy as a predictor of survival in patients with end-stage liver disease. Liver Transpl 2007;13: 1366–71.
12. Bajaj JS, Schubert CM, Heuman DM, et al. Persistence of cognitive impairment after resolution of overt hepatic encephalopathy. Gastroenterology 2010;138(7): 2332–40.

13. Bajaj JS, Schubert CM, Sanyal AJ, et al. Severity of chronic cognitive impairment in cirrhosis increases with number of episodes of overt hepatic encephalopathy. J Hepatol 2010;52(Suppl 1):S66.
14. Fichet J, Mercier E, Genee O, et al. Prognosis and 1-year mortality of intensive care unit patients with severe hepatic encephalopathy. J Crit Care 2009;24:364–70.
15. Conn HO, Lieberthal MM. The hepatic coma syndromes and lactulose. Baltimore (MD): Williams & Wilkins; 1979.
16. Cordoba J, Blei AT. Hepatic encephalopathy. In: Schiff ER, Sorrell MF, Maddrey WC, editors. Schiff's diseases of the liver, vol. 1, 10th edition. Philadelphia: Lippincott Williams &Wilkins; 2007. p. 569–99.
17. Hassanein T, Blei AT, Perry W, et al. Performance of the hepatic encephalopathy scoring algorithm in a clinical trial of patients with cirrhosis and severe hepatic encephalopathy. Am J Gastroenterol 2009;104:1392–400.
18. Williams R, James OF, Morgan MY. Evaluation of the efficacy and safety of rifaximin in the treatment of hepatic encephalopathy: a double-blind, randomized, dose-finding multi-centre study. Eur J Gastroenterol Hepatol 2000;12:203–8.
19. Conn HO, Leevy CM, Vlahcevic ZR, et al. Comparison of lactulose and neomycin in the treatment of chronic portal-systemic-encephalopathy: a double blind controlled trial. Gastroenterology 1977;72:573–83.
20. Blei AT, Cordoba J, Practice Parameters Committee of the American College of Gastroenterology. Hepatic encephalopathy. Am J Gastroenterol 2001;96:1968–76.
21. Riordan SM, Williams R. Treatment of hepatic encephalopathy. N Engl J Med 1997;337(7):473–9.
22. Munoz SJ. Hepatic encephalopathy. Med Clin North Am 2008;92:795–812.
23. Caruana P, Shah N. Hepatic encephalopathy: are NH_4 levels and protein restriction obsolete? Pract Gastroenterol 2011;95:6–18.
24. Morgan MY, Blei A, Grungreiff K, et al. The treatment of hepatic encephalopathy. Metab Brain Dis 2007;22:389–405.
25. Als-Nielsen B, Gluud LL, Gluud C. Non-absorbable disaccharides for hepatic encephalopathy:systematic review of randomized trials. BMJ 2004;328:1046.
26. Bass NM, Mullen KD, Sanyal A, et al. Rifaximin treatment in hepatic encephalopathy. N Engl J Med 2010;362:1071–81.
27. Kanematsu T, Koyanagi N, Matsumata T, et al. Lack of preventive effect of branched-chain amino acid solution on postoperative hepatic encephalopathy in patients with cirrhosis: a randomized, prospective trial. Surgery 1988;104(3):482–8.
28. Hassanein TI, Tofteng F, Brown RS Jr, et al. Randomized controlled study of extracorporeal albumin dialysis for hepatic encephalopathy in advanced cirrhosis. Hepatology 2007;46:1853–62.
29. Sharma BC, Sharma P, Agrawal A, et al. Secondary prophylaxis of hepatic encephalopathy: an open label randomized controlled trial of lactulose versus placebo. Gastroenterology 2009;137:885–91.
30. Rolachon A, Zarski JP, Lutz JM, et al. Is the intestinal lavage with a solution of mannitol effective in the prevention of post-hemorrhagic hepatic encephalopathy in patients with liver cirrhosis? results of a randomized prospective study. Gastroenterol Clin Biol 1994;18(12):1057–62.
31. Uribe M, Campollo O, Vargas F, et al. Acidifying enemas (lactitol and lactose) vs. nonacidifying enemas (tap water) to treat acute portal-systemic encephalopathy: a double-blind, randomized clinical trial. Hepatology 1987;7(4):639–43.
32. Kircheis G, Nilius R, Held C, et al. Therapeutic efficacy of L-ornithine-L-aspartate infusions in patients with cirrhosis and hepatic encephalopathy: results of a placebo-controlled, double-blind study. Hepatology 1997;25(6):1351–60.

33. Stauch S, Kircheis G, Adler G, et al. Oral L-ornithine-L-aspartate therapy of chronic hepatic encephalopathy: results of a placebo-controlled double-blind study. J Hepatol 1998;28(5):856–64.
34. Sushma S, Dasarathy S, Tandon RK, et al. Sodium benzoate in the treatment of acute hepatic encephalopathy: a double-blind randomized trial. Hepatology 1992;16(1):138–44.
35. Reding P, Duchateau J, Bataille C. Oral zinc supplementation improves hepatic encephalopathy. Results of a randomized controlled trial. Lancet 1984;2(8401): 493–5.
36. Riggio O, Ariosto F, Merli M, et al. Short-term oral zinc supplementation does not improve chronic hepatic encephalopathy. Results of a double-blind crossover trial. Dig Dis Sci 1991;36(9):1204–8.
37. Sotil EU, Gottstein J, Ayala E, et al. Impact of preoperative overt hepatic enceph-alopathy on neurocognitive function after liver transplantation. Liver Transpl 2009; 15:184–92.
38. Bass NM. Review article the current pharmacological therapies for hepatic encephalopathy. Aliment Pharmacol Ther 2007;25(Suppl 1):23–31.
39. Devrajani BR, Shah SZ, Devrajani T, et al. Precipitating factors of hepatic enceph-alopathy at a tertiary care hospital Jamshoro, Hyderabad. J Pak Med Assoc 2009;59:683–6.
40. Strauss E, Gomes de Sa Ribeiro Mde F. Bacterial infections associated with hepatic encephalopathy: prevalence and outcome. Ann Hepatol 2003;2:41–5.
41. Zushi S, Imai Y, Fukuda K, et al. Endoscopic coagulation therapy is successful for improving encephalopathy in cirrhotic patients with gastric antral vascular ecta-sia. Dig Endosc 2005;17:32–5.
42. Jalan R, Kapoor D. Enhanced renal ammonia excretion following volume expan-sion in patients with well compensated cirrhosis of the liver. Gut 2003;52:1041–5.
43. Pockros P, Hassanein T, Vierling J, et al. Phase 2, multicenter, randomized study of AST-120 (spherical carbon adsorbent) vs. lactulose in the treatment of low-grade hepatic encephalopathy. J Hepatol 2009;50(Suppl 1):S43–4.
44. Kramer L, Tribl B, Gendo A, et al. Partial pressure of ammonia versus ammonia in hepatic encephalopathy. Hepatology 2000;31:30–4.
45. Ong JP, Aggarwal A, Krieger D, et al. Correlation between ammonia levels and the severity of hepatic encephalopathy. Am J Med 2003;114:188–93.
46. Plauth M, Roske AE, Romaniuk P, et al. Post-feeding hyperammonaemia in patients with transjugular intrahepatic portosystemic shunt and liver cirrhosis: role of small intestinal ammonia release and route of nutrient administration. Gut 2000;46:849–55.
47. Weissenborn K, Tietge UJ, Bokemeyer M, et al. Liver transplantation improves hepatic myelopathy: evidence by three cases. Gastroenterology 2003;124: 346–51.
48. Als-Nielsen B, Gluud LL, Gluud C. Nonabsorbable disaccharides for hepatic encephalopathy. Cochrane Database Syst Rev 2004;2:CD003044.
49. Lukers B, Nierman DM, Schiano TD. Lactulose: how many ways can one drug be prescribed? Am J Gastroenterol 2011;106(9):1726–7.
50. Bass N. Treatment of patients with hepatic encephalopathy: review of the latest data from EASL 2011. Gastroenterol Hepatol 2011;7(Suppl 9):1–15.
51. Malaguarnera M, Gargante MP, Malaguarnera G, et al. Bifidobacterium combined with fructo-oligosaccharide versus lactulose in the treatment of patients with hepatic encephalopathy. Eur J Gastroenterol Hepatol 2010;22: 199–206.

52. Iwasa M, Nakao M, Kato Y, et al. Dietary fiber decreases ammonia levels in patients with cirrhosis. Hepatology 2005;41:217–8 [author reply: 219].

53. Liu Q, Duan ZP, Ha DK, et al. Synbiotic modulation of gut flora: effect on minimal hepatic encephalopathy in patients with cirrhosis. Hepatology 2004;39:1441–9.

54. Seyan AS, Hughes RD, Shawcross DL. Changing face of hepatic encephalopathy: role of inflammation and oxidative stress. World J Gastroenterol 2010;16:3347–57.

55. Gentile S, Guarino G, Romano M, et al. A randomized controlled trial of acarbose in hepatic encephalopathy. Clin Gastroenterol Hepatol 2005;3:184–91.

56. Gerard L, Garey KW, DuPont HL. Rifaximin: a nonabsorbable rifamycin antibiotic for use in nonsystemic gastrointestinal infections. Expert Rev Anti Infect Ther 2005;3:201–11.

57. Jiang ZD, DuPont HL. Rifaximin: in vitro and in vivo antibacterial activity—a review. Chemotherapy 2005;51(Suppl 1):67–72.

58. Debbia EA, Maioli E, Roveta S, et al. Effects of rifaximin on bacterial virulence mechanisms at supra-and sub-inhibitory concentrations. J Chemother 2008;20:186–94.

59. Sanyal A, Younossi ZM, Bass NM, et al. Randomised clinical trial: rifaximin improves health-related quality of life in cirrhotic patients with hepatic encephalopathy—a double-blind placebo-controlled study. Aliment Pharmacol Ther 2011;34(8):853–61. [Epub ahead of print].

60. Sanyal A, Bass N, Mullen K, et al. Rifaximin treatment improved quality of life in patients with hepatic encephalopathy: results of a large, randomized, placebo-controlled trial. J Hepatol 2010;52(Suppl 1):S7.

61. Mullen KD, Poordad F, Rossaro L, et al. Long term efficacy and survival in patients treated with the gut-selective antibiotic rifaximin (550 mg BID) for the maintenance of remission from overt hepatic encephalopathy. Gastroenterol Hepatol 2011;7(6 Suppl 9):1–15.

62. Vlachogiannakos K, Viazis N, Vasianopoulou P, et al. Long-term administration of rifaximin improves the prognosis of patients with alcohol-related decompensated cirrhosis: a case-control study. Berlin, Germany: EASL; 2011. poster.

63. Leise MD, Pedersen R, Kamath PS, et al. Impact of rifaximin treatment on survival in patients with end-stage liver disease. Hepatology 2010;52(Suppl 1):331A.

64. Jiang Q, Jiang G, Welty TE, et al. Naloxone in the management of hepatic encephalopathy. J Clin Pharm Ther 2010;35:333–41.

65. Als-Nielsen B, Gluud LL, Gluud C. Benzodiazepine receptor antagonists for hepatic encephalopathy. Cochrane Database Syst Rev 2004;2:CD002798.

66. Basu P, Shah NJ, Krishnaswamy N, et al. Transdermal rivastigmine for treatment of encephalopathy in liver cirrhosis—a randomized placebo controlled trial (TREC TRIAL). J Hepatol 2010;52(Suppl 1):S67–8.

67. Cordoba J, Lopez-Hellin J, Planas M, et al. Normal protein diet for episodic hepatic encephalopathy: results of a randomized study. J Hepatol 2004;41:38–43.

68. Bajaj JS. Review article: the modern management of hepatic encephalopathy. Aliment Pharmacol Ther 2010;31(5):537–47.

69. Balzola F, Sanna C, Ottobrelli A, et al. Chronic hepatic encephalopathy (HE) in patients with severe liver cirrhosis: efficacy of the wheat and milk protein free diet in the reduction of clinical episodes. Gastroenterol Hepatol 2011;7(6 Suppl 9):1–15.

70. Takuma Y, Nouso K, Makino Y, et al. Clinical trial: oral zinc in hepatic encephalopathy. Aliment Pharmacol Ther 2010;32:1080–90.

71. Jiang Q, Jiang XH, Zheng MH, et al. L-ornithine-l-aspartate in the management of hepatic encephalopathy: a meta-analysis. J Gastroenterol Hepatol 2009;24:9–14.
72. Ocera therapeutics completes first in human studies with OCR-002 for the treatment of hyperammonemia and hepatic encephalopathy. San Diego (CA): Ocera; 2010.
73. Als-Nielsen B, Koretz RL, Kjaergard L, et al. Branched-chain amino acids for hepatic encephalopathy. Cochrane Database Syst Rev 2003;2:CD001939.
74. Malaguarnera M, Vacante M, Motta M, et al. Acetyl-L-carnitine improves cognitive functions in severe hepatic encephalopathy: a randomized and controlled clinical trial. Metab Brain Dis 2011;26(4):281–9.
75. Riggio O, Masini A, Efrati C, et al. Pharmacological prophylaxis of hepatic encephalopathy after transjugular intrahepatic portosystemic shunt: a randomized controlled study. J Hepatol 2005;42(5):674–9.

Management of Covert Hepatic Encephalopathy

Kevin D. Mullen, MD, FRCPI*, Ravi K. Prakash, MBBS, MD, MRCP (UK)

KEYWORDS

- Hepatic encephalopathy • Covert hepatic encephalopathy
- Minimal hepatic encephalopathy
- Psychometric hepatic encephalopathy score

Until recently, most physicians did not give any consideration to treating what was called minimal hepatic encephalopathy (HE). It was defined and detected in patients but the word, *minimal*, implied that the consequences of treating minimal HE were insignificant. Considerable data now exist to contradict this perspective. Employability,[1,2] driving capacity,[3,4] and many domains of health-related quality of life[5–7] are reduced in patients with minimal HE. Moreover, once minimal HE is identified, more than 50% of patients develop overt HE within 30 months.[8] Now that minimal HE has been shown associated with consequences, it has been decided to change its name to covert HE.[9] This article discusses the criteria for diagnosis of covert HE; the term, *covert HE*, is now officially endorsed by the International Society for Hepatic Encephalopathy and Nitrogen Metabolism (ISHEN).

One of the barriers to diagnosing covert HE has been the lack of availability of validated tools to detect/measure covert HE. The psychometric hepatic encephalopathy score (PHES) was officially endorsed for the detection of covert (then called subclinical and later called minimal) HE and remains so today.[10] The battery of psychometric tests was originally developed by Schomerus and Hamster[11] and modified later by Weissenborn and colleagues.[12] The tested populations were nonalcoholic cirrhotics versus controls residing in Europe. The PHES is used widely in Europe but copyright measures and lack of normative controls in the United States have hindered the adoption of this gold standard test system in the United States.[13] Most reports on psychometric test detection of covert HE came from large European medical centers with plenty of staff to administer psychometric tests. Some medical centers in the United States associated with liver transplant units have adopted other testing systems as well as other versions of PHES to diagnose covert HE.[14] Many cirrhotic patients with covert HE, however, are outside liver transplant centers and are generally seen

Division of Gastroenterology, MetroHealth Medical Center, Case Western Reserve University, 2500 MetroHealth Drive, Cleveland, OH 44109, USA
* Corresponding author.
E-mail address: kevin.mullen@case.edu

Clin Liver Dis 16 (2012) 91–93
doi:10.1016/j.cld.2011.12.006
1089-3261/12/$ – see front matter © 2012 Published by Elsevier Inc.

by individual practitioners. Therefore, there is a premium in the United States for developing simple-to-use testing system for the detection of covert HE. Once this occurs, one of the major barriers in the management of covert HE will be overcome.

The final obstacle to management of covert HE is the absence of cost-effectiveness data to support routine treatment of covert HE. There are data showing improvement in quality of life[6,7] and driving capacity[15] along with improved performance in psychometric tests, including the inhibitory control test with current HE therapies, such as lactulose and rifaximin. Better still, most of these trials are placebo controlled, thus avoiding all the problems with overt HE treatment where placebo arms for treatment trials were thought to be unethical.[16] The treatment of patients at risk for recurrent bouts of overt HE is justifiable based on preventing or reducing hospitalizations. The cost issues are more difficult to reconcile with the reversal of minimal or covert HE primarily because it is difficult to estimate the costs of reducing quality of life, poor driving capacity, and other aspects associated with covert HE.

Once a totally standardized set of criteria is used worldwide to diagnose and measure covert HE, cost-effectiveness data will be generated quickly. The adoption of the PHES system stimulated a great deal of productive research once physicians were able to use the same tools to diagnose covert HE. The only problem that arose was the general lack of availability of tests for independent nonacademic center–based physicians. A system that can be used as a computer-accessible scoring algorithm would a greeted with great enthusiasm by clinicians if the cost of the testing system were reasonable or reimbursed through health care agencies. The current inhibitory control tests that have been validated and championed by Jasmohan Bajaj for several years are available online free of charge.[17] Whether others use it with the accuracy and reproducibility of this group remains to be determined.

REFERENCES

1. Schomerus H, Hamster W. Quality of life in cirrhotics with minimal hepatic encephalopathy. Metab Brain Dis 2001;16(1–2):37–41.
2. Bajaj JS. Minimal hepatic encephalopathy matters in daily life. World J Gastroenterol 2008;14(23):3609–15.
3. Bajaj JS, Hafeezullah M, Hoffmann RG, et al. Minimal hepatic encephalopathy: a vehicle for accidents and traffic violations. Am J Gastroenterol 2007;102(9): 1903–9.
4. Kircheis G, Knoche A, Hilger N, et al. Hepatic encephalopathy and fitness to drive. Gastroenterology 2009;137(5):1706–15, e1–9.
5. Groeneweg M, Quero JC, De Bruijn I, et al. Subclinical hepatic encephalopathy impairs daily functioning. Hepatology 1998;28(1):45–9.
6. Prasad S, Dhiman RK, Duseja A, et al. Lactulose improves cognitive functions and health-related quality of life in patients with cirrhosis who have minimal hepatic encephalopathy. Hepatology 2007;45(3):549–59.
7. Sidhu SS, Goyal O, Mishra BP, et al. Rifaximin improves psychometric performance and health-related quality of life in patients with minimal hepatic encephalopathy (the RIME Trial). Am J Gastroenterol 2011;106(2):307–16.
8. Bustamante J, Rimola A, Ventura PJ, et al. Prognostic significance of hepatic encephalopathy in patients with cirrhosis. J Hepatol 1999;30(5):890–5.
9. Bajaj JS, Cordoba J, Mullen KD, et al. Review article: the design of clinical trials in hepatic encephalopathy—an International Society for Hepatic Encephalopathy and Nitrogen Metabolism (ISHEN) consensus statement. Aliment Pharmacol Ther 2011;33(7):739–47.

10. Ferenci P, Lockwood A, Mullen K, et al. Hepatic encephalopathy—definition, nomenclature, diagnosis, and quantification: final report of the working party at the 11th World Congresses of Gastroenterology, Vienna, 1998. Hepatology 2002;35(3):716–21.
11. Schomerus H, Hamster W. Neuropsychological aspects of portal-systemic encephalopathy. Metab Brain Dis 1998;13(4):361–77.
12. Weissenborn K, Ennen JC, Schomerus H, et al. Neuropsychological characterization of hepatic encephalopathy. J Hepatol 2001;34(5):768–73.
13. Iduru S, Mullen KD. The demise of the pencil? New computer-assisted tests for minimal hepatic encephalopathy. Gastroenterology 2008;135(5):1455–6.
14. Prakash R, Mullen KD. Mechanisms, diagnosis and management of hepatic encephalopathy. Nat Rev Gastroenterol Hepatol 2010;7(9):515–25.
15. Bajaj JS, Heuman DM, Wade JB, et al. Rifaximin improves driving simulator performance in a randomized trial of patients with minimal hepatic encephalopathy. Gastroenterology 2011;140(2):478–487.e1.
16. Mullen KD, Amodio P, Morgan MY. Therapeutic studies in hepatic encephalopathy. Metab Brain Dis 2007;22(3–4):407–23.
17. Available at: http://www.hecme.tv. Accessed December 24, 2011.

Malnutrition in Cirrhosis: Contribution and Consequences of Sarcopenia on Metabolic and Clinical Responses

Pranav Periyalwar, MD[a,b], Srinivasan Dasarathy, MD[b,c],*

KEYWORDS

• Malnutrition • Cirrhosis • Sarcopenia • Metabolism

Cirrhosis with portosystemic shunting is associated with malnutrition, which is the most frequent, yet potentially reversible complication that worsens with disease progression and adversely affects outcome in these patients.[1-5] Malnutrition in cirrhosis is associated with major complications that include sepsis, uncontrolled ascites, hepatic encephalopathy (HE), spontaneous bacterial peritonitis, and hepatorenal syndrome that develop in 65% of malnourished patients versus 12% of well-nourished patients.[4,6-10] Several recent reviews have discussed the current clinical problems and therapy for malnutrition in cirrhosis.[11-13] However, the major limitation of these is the lack of focus on the recent advances and potentially exciting data from diverse fields besides hepatology. This review focuses on the current understanding of malnutrition and the newer molecular pathways and targets that are likely to result in novel and specific therapies to reverse its components. Malnutrition in cirrhosis consists of a loss of skeletal muscle and adipose tissue mass. Even though it is being recognized that this combination should be defined as cachexia,[14,15] the

---

[a] Department of Gastroenterology, Metrohealth Medical Center, 2500 Metrohealth Drive, Cleveland, OH 44109, USA
[b] Department of Gastroenterology and Hepatology, Lerner Research Institute, Cleveland Clinic, 9500 Euclid Avenue, NE4-208, Cleveland, OH 44195, USA
[c] Department of Pathobiology, Lerner Research Institute, Cleveland Clinic, 9500 Euclid Avenue, NE4-208, Cleveland, OH 44195, USA
* Corresponding author. Department of Gastroenterology and Hepatology, Lerner Research Institute, Cleveland Clinic, 9500 Euclid Avenue, NE4-208, Cleveland, OH 44195.
E-mail address: dasaras@ccf.org

Clin Liver Dis 16 (2012) 95–131
doi:10.1016/j.cld.2011.12.009
1089-3261/12/$ – see front matter © 2012 Elsevier Inc. All rights reserved.

predominant loss of muscle mass in cirrhosis suggests that sarcopenia or loss of skeletal muscle mass is the primary nutritional consequence.[16,17] In patients with cirrhosis, the prevalence of malnutrition characterized by loss of lean body mass and diminished skeletal muscle weight is estimated to be between 20% to 60% in different studies.[5,18–21] Most studies have focused on quantifying lean body mass using different instruments, but the skeletal muscle constitutes between 40% and 50% of the lean body mass.[22] More precise measures of skeletal muscle mass that are being recognized are the direct measures using imaging techniques.[16,17] Skeletal muscle loss in cirrhosis worsens with advancing severity of liver disease as measured by Child's score and the development of portosystemic shunting.[19,23–25] There has been limited success using several nutritional and other interventions in reversing malnutrition and low skeletal muscle mass in cirrhosis.[1,2,23,26,27] Only partial improvement in anthropometric measures and body weight occur when enteral nutrition or parenteral amino acid mixtures are given.[28,29] Neither recombinant growth hormone nor insulinlike growth factor 1 (IGF1) in human and animal models of cirrhosis were able to result in complete recovery of skeletal muscle mass.[30–32] These poor results are likely related to the limited understanding of the pathophysiologic mechanisms responsible for diminished muscle mass in cirrhosis and portosystemic shunting.[1,33] Several factors may contribute to this and include the predominantly descriptive nature of the human studies, heterogeneity in the definitions for malnutrition, limited mechanistic studies on skeletal muscle loss in cirrhosis, and the preponderance of publications on skeletal muscle biology in nonliver journals.[34,35] Despite the number of publications in this area, there are few studies that have reconciled the recent and exciting data obtained from studies on skeletal muscle biology into our current understanding of malnutrition in cirrhosis.[22,36] The present review aims toward integrating our current understanding of the clinical consequences, mechanisms, and therapeutic targets and approaches toward reversing the major complication of cirrhosis, sarcopenia, or loss of skeletal muscle mass.

Recent studies in animal models and cell culture systems have contributed significantly to our understanding of potential mechanisms responsible for sarcopenia in portosystemic shunting in cirrhosis.[37–42]

Our understanding of the metabolic processes in cirrhosis, skeletal muscle, and whole body protein, fat, and carbohydrate metabolism has increased over the past 2 decades, during which time liver transplantation has become a viable and definitive treatment option for end-stage liver disease. Several questions, however, remain unanswered. These include the precise definition of malnutrition in cirrhosis; prevalence of malnutrition in cirrhosis that is affected by the method used to define malnutrition; the impact of malnutrition on outcome before, during, and after liver transplantation; the available therapeutic options; and the outcome in response to these interventions. Additionally, recent exciting and novel data from the authors' laboratory, and that of others, to identify the role of molecular signaling pathways are expected to provide novel insights into the management of patients with cirrhosis.[36,43]

MALNUTRITION IN LIVER DISEASE: DEFINITIONS

There is wide heterogeneity in the definition of malnutrition in cirrhosis, primarily because adult malnutrition is not well defined. In children, malnutrition is clearly defined as predominantly protein malnutrition or kwashiorkor and combined protein and calorie malnutrition or marasmus. In humans, most proteins are located in the skeletal muscle,[44–47] and we have, therefore, defined clinical adult protein malnutrition as primarily skeletal muscle loss. Energy malnutrition is more difficult to define clearly, but because adipose tissue is the largest repository of calories, adult fat malnutrition can be defined as a reduction in whole body fat mass. Loss of skeletal muscle mass is also known as sarcopenia, even though this term has traditionally been used to define loss of muscle mass with aging.[14,15] More recently, other terms have been used that include cachexia, which is defined as loss of both muscle and fat mass that is not responsive to providing adequate dietary intake, and precachexia, which is based on the percentile values of the measured muscle and fat mass compared with controls.[14,15] However, it must be reiterated that these consensus definitions are being developed, but their relevance to the complex metabolic and nutritional derangements in cirrhosis have not been evaluated. It may, however, be summarized that based on our current understanding, malnutrition in cirrhosis comprises reduced muscle mass and strength, called sarcopenia, as well as loss of subcutaneous and visceral fat mass that may be called *adipopenia*. The term hepatic cachexia can be used to define the proportionate loss of both muscle and adipose tissue mass. Finally, the rapid increase in prevalence of fatty liver–related cirrhosis is increasing the number of patients who have sarcopenic obesity characterized by a disproportionate loss of skeletal muscle mass with preserved or increased visceral or subcutaneous adipose tissue mass. Given these reasons, it may be best to avoid the term, malnutrition in cirrhosis, because it can be used to refer to sarcopenia, adipopenia, cachexia, precachexia, obesity, sarcopenic obesity, and micronutrient deficiencies. Precision in definition will permit a clear definition of the patient population being studied and the outcome measures being quantified. Given the lack of such a consensus definition in patients with cirrhosis, the authors have defined these terms in the specific population of patients with cirrhosis (**Table 1**).

METHODS TO ASSESS MALNUTRITION IN CIRRHOSIS

As previously stated, most publications on malnutrition in cirrhosis use heterogeneous definitions. Standard nutritional assessment instruments use laboratory tests, such as prothrombin time; albumin; prealbumin; transferrin; creatinine height index; and on tests of immune function, such as the delayed-type hypersensitivity reactions.[48–50] Because end-stage liver disease or cirrhosis confound the common measures of nutritional status, their utility in these patients is reduced. Patients with cirrhosis have significant impairment in their hepatic synthetic function that results in low serum albumin, prealbumin, transferrin levels, and prolonged prothrombin time. These levels will result in an overestimation of the prevalence of malnutrition in these patients.[51,52] Renal impairment is common in cirrhosis, making the creatinine height index an imprecise measure of malnutrition.[53] Anthropometric measures are affected by altered fluid status caused by ascites, peripheral edema, diuretic and salt intake, and concomitant rental failure that makes weight changes difficult to interpret.[54,55] Skinfold thickness that measures subcutaneous fat mass, upper-arm measure of muscle area (midarm muscle area), and subjective global assessment (SGA) has additional limitations, including interobserver variability.[56,57] Furthermore, with the change in demographics and socioeconomic patterns, there are changes in the normal values, and concurrent norms should be used for defining criteria for sarcopenia and cachexia.[58] Finally, the anergy in cirrhosis makes delayed-type hypersensitivity an inaccurate gauge of malnutrition.[51,59]

Several indirect, in vivo methods have been used to quantify body composition in cirrhosis. These methods include total-body electrical conductivity, bioelectrical impedance, dual energy x-ray absorptiometry, deuterium dilution, air displacement plethysmography, and magnetic resonance spectroscopy.[60–62] These methods are

Table 1
Prevalence of malnutrition in cirrhosis

Author/Year	n	Definition of Malnutrition	Prevalence (%)	Cause of Cirrhosis
Alberino et al,[19] 2001	212	TSF MAMA	Severe 34 Moderate 20	Alcohol Viral
Akerman et al,[59] 1993	104	TSF <fifth percentile MAMC <fifth percentile	33 <fifth percentile 43	Alcohol Viral Primary biliary Sclerosing cholangitis
Alvares-da-silva & Reverbel da,[4] 2005	50	SGA Prognostic nutritional state Handgrip strength	28 18 63	All causes
Figueiredo et al,[74] 2005	79	Body cell mass TBF	31.6	Alcohol Viral
Caly et al,[71] 2003	77	TSF Albumin	71	Alcohol Viral
Caregaro et al,[72] 1996	120	Anthropometric Visceral	34 81	Alcohol Viral
de Carvalho et al,[76] 2010	300	Anthropometric	75	All causes
Lehnert et al,[75] 2001	50	BIA$_{BCM}$ TBF	Child A, 71 Child C, 81	Viral Primary biliary Autoimmune
Hasse et al,[49] 1993	20	Immunologic SGA, moderate SGA, severe	59 70 15	Viral Primary biliary Wilson disease
Hehir et al,[77] 1985	13	Anergy Lymphocyte Albumin	58 92 62	All causes
Loguercio et al,[78] 1996	184	Skinfold thickness	Child A, 8 Child B/C, 26	All causes

Mendenhall et al,[68] 1984	363	Clinical diagnosis	100	Alcohol Viral
Mills et al,[79] 1983	30	DTH Vitamin deficiency MAMC	29 43 13	Alcohol Viral
Morgan et al,[65] 1996	60	Anthropometric BIA$_{BCM}$	29	Alcohol Viral Primary biliary Autoimmune
Peng et al,[18] 2007	268	Indirect calorimetry Grip strength	51	All causes
Reisman et al,[80] 1997	1015	Clinical nutritional state	33–60	Alcohol Viral Primary biliary Autoimmune
Roongpisuthipong et al,[73] 2001	60	Visceral protein DTH Ideal body weight	45 22 13.3	Alcohol Viral
Sam and Nguyen,[81] 2009	114,703	Clinical diagnosis	6.1 (1.9 control)	Alcohol Viral Primary biliary Autoimmune
Tai et al,[82] 2010	36	MAMC SGA	50 40	Alcohol Viral Primary biliary Sclerosing cholangitis

Abbreviations: BIA$_{BCM}$, bioelectrical impedance analyzer measured body cell mass; BIA$_{TBP}$ bioelectrical impedance analyzer measured total body protein; BMI, body mass index; SGA, subjective global assessment; TBF, total body fat; TBP, total body protein; TSF, triceps skinfold thickness.

Summary: Eighteen studies, with a total of 3041 of subjects enrolled, measure malnutrition by a variety of methods, including SGA, MAMC, TSF, BIA, and clinical assessment. The prevalence of malnutrition ranges from 6.1% to 100.0%. Cause of cirrhosis included alcohol, viral, primary biliary, autoimmune, sclerosing cholangitis, and Wilson disease.

based on the principle that at least 2 components exist in the body fat mass and fat-free mass that is essentially water, protein, and mineral.[63] By determining the whole body weight and fat mass, it is assumed that the remaining weight is nonfat or lean mass. Because 40% to 60% of lean body mass in humans and rodents is contributed by skeletal muscle mass, quantification of lean body or fat-free mass is considered to be a measure of whole body skeletal muscle mass.[64] There are also concerns expressed about the 2-compartment model obtained from these studies, and alternative 3-component and 4-component models have been proposed.[63,65–67] These multicomponent models suffer from limitations in cirrhosis because of the alteration in hydration, bone mineralization, and fluid shifts. Hence, there seems to be no true gold standard or reference technique to quantify malnutrition in cirrhosis. The choice of application is based on cost, logistics, availability, and the need for accuracy and segmental body composition. Based on published studies on malnutrition, the authors' definitions of protein malnutrition to be reflected by skeletal muscle mass and fat malnutrition quantified by the loss of subcutaneous and visceral fat mass as well as altered thermogenesis seem most clinically relevant and can be applied at the bedside.

Recently, psoas muscle area quantified on a single section of computed tomography (CT) of the abdomen at the L3/4 level has been validated as a reliable, noninvasive measure of reduced whole body skeletal muscle mass in cirrhosis.[16,17] The authors have observed this to be equally reliable for quantifying visceral fat mass on the same section. Because CT of the abdomen is routinely used to screen for lesions in patients with cirrhosis, this can also be used to quantify skeletal muscle and fat mass in these patients. Despite its simplicity, cost and irradiation are 2 considerations that need to be taken into account when using this method.

PREVALENCE OF MALNUTRITION IN CIRRHOSIS

A high prevalence of malnutrition has been reported in patients with cirrhosis in studies in which visceral protein status and immunologic measures are included in the nutritional assessment.[48,68,69] The prevalence of nutritional disorders is lower when malnutrition is diagnosed by anthropometric measures only.[54,55] Differences in the cause and severity of disease also affect the estimated prevalence of malnutrition in cirrhosis.[48,70–73] A review of studies published that examined the prevalence of malnutrition using defined criteria is shown in **Table 1**.[4,18,19,49,59,65,68,71–82] It can be summarized from these data that the prevalence of malnutrition depends primarily on the definition chosen, cause of the liver disease, the stage of the disease, and the methods used to quantify malnutrition. Anthropometric measures have been considered to be most dependable; using only these criteria, the prevalence is significantly lower than previously estimated. The lowest estimate from the largest study in 114,703 hospitalized patients with cirrhosis compared with hospitalized patients without cirrhosis showed a prevalence of 6.1% in cirrhosis compared with 1.9% in controls.[81] The major limitation of this study is that malnutrition was diagnosed imprecisely based on a clinical discharge diagnosis. The investigators acknowledge the limitations but suggest that their data support previous published literature on the high (more than 4 fold) prevalence of malnutrition in cirrhosis compared with patients without cirrhosis. Other studies have confirmed that using a combination of biochemical and immunologic studies overestimates the prevalence of muscle and fat loss as estimated by clinical and anthropometric methods.[19,72] Given these observations, it would be appropriate to have a standardized method of assessment of protein and fat malnutrition in cirrhosis. An extensive review of the data suggests that the modified SGA that is appropriate in cirrhosis and precise upper-extremity anthropometric measures may be the best available option.[4,49] A recent study by the authors' group in 97 hospitalized patients has shown that grip strength and SGA remain the most feasible instruments in assessing the nutritional status and outcome.

These data suggest that based on the definition of the specific component of malnutrition, an appropriate measurement instrument should be chosen. Increasing interest in imaging methods is because of the ability to distinguish the reduction of skeletal muscle and visceral and adipose tissue mass. However, functional measures of muscle strength remain one of the most relevant measures of sarcopenia.[83]

SEVERITY OF LIVER DISEASE WORSENS SARCOPENIA

Malnutrition has also been related to the severity of liver disease as estimated by Child's score.[73] Several modifications of the original Child's score have been used, including the Child-Turcotte, Campbell Child, and Pugh-Child scoring systems.[80] In the Pugh modification, the nutritional status was replaced by prothrombin time; the rationale for this was that the nutritional assessment used in the other versions had a significant subjective evaluation, whereas the prothrombin time in combination with serum albumin provides a more objective measure of long-term nutritional evaluation.[84] However, as has been discussed earlier, these are truly measures of hepatic function and are likely to show greater abnormality with worsening severity of liver disease. The authors have specifically excluded those investigators who used the Child-Turcotte and Campbell Child scoring system because these have nutritional evaluation incorporated into them and are, therefore, biased in favor of a higher prevalence of malnutrition in advanced disease. In 3 published studies that evaluated the impact of severity of underlying liver disease as measured by the Child-Pugh scoring system showed that there is evidence of malnutrition as assessed by grip strength, body cell mass, body fat mass, and ideal body weight early in the course of the disease.[73,74,85] These measures of nutritional deficiency become worse with progressive severity of liver disease.[73,74,85] Other measures of severity of liver disease, including the model for end-stage liver disease (MELD) score, have not been systematically assessed for their relation to the severity of sarcopenia, cachexia, or malnutrition.

These observations suggest that clinical and anthropometric measures of loss of muscle mass and fat mass are common in cirrhosis and worsen with the progression of liver disease.

CLINICAL IMPLICATIONS OF MALNUTRITION IN CIRRHOSIS

For practical clinical purposes, the impact of malnutrition in cirrhosis on outcome can be examined by the effect of skeletal muscle loss on survival and complications of cirrhosis. With the availability of liver transplantation, aggressive intensive care, antibiotics, renal support, and endoscopic interventions to prevent and treat the complications of cirrhosis, there is a resurgence of interest in the nutritional management of these patients. Several studies have consistently shown that malnutrition in cirrhosis affects the survival and the development of the complications of cirrhosis.

Malnutrition and Survival in Cirrhosis

Several investigators have examined the impact of malnutrition, primarily using instruments that measure sarcopenia, and observed that worsening severity of muscle loss is accompanied by higher mortality (**Table 2**).[3–5,10,16,17,76,86–91] It is interesting that despite a large number of studies across the world demonstrating that sarcopenia

Table 2
Impact of malnutrition on survival in cirrhosis

Author/Year	n	Pretransplant Malnutrition (%)	Posttransplant Survival
Alvares-da-Silva & Reverbel da,[4] 2005	50	SGA 28 PNI 19 HG 63	20.7% mortality in subjects with PCM vs 0% without PCM, assessed by HG; $P > .05$ for HG vs other variables; 21.4% mortality in subjects with PCM vs 8.3% without PCM, assessed by SGA; $P > .05$; 0% mortality with and without PCM when assessed by PNI; $P > .05$
Bathgate et al,[86] 1999	121	53	In malnourished patients (TSF <fifth percentile) compared with well nourished, acute rejection occurred in 53% vs 35%; $P = .97$; comparing malnourished based on MAMC <fifth percentile to well nourished 15% vs 64% had acute rejection; $P = .01$
Bilbao et al,[3] 2003	55	50	Mortality rate of 46% for patients with liver resection and 36% for patients with liver transplant; Median survival was 85 mo in both groups, and 1-, 5-, and 10-y actuarial survival after LR and LT was 92% and 78%, 70% and 65%, and 50% and 60%, respectively ($P = .8$); Pretransplant renal insufficiency is the most significant risk factor for early mortality
de Carvalho et al,[76] 2010	70	69	PCM was significantly increased in patients with cirrhosis compared with patients without cirrhosis at 90 d based on pretransplant PCM score (OR: 53.4, CI: 1.9–1481.9, $P = .019$) and 1 y after transplant based on TSF (OR: 7.202, CI: 1.2–44.1, $P = .033$)
Deschenes et al,[87] 1997	109	33	6-mo survival rates for patients classified as Child-Pugh A, B, C were 90%, 78%, and 65%; No 6-mo survival impact of nutritional status
Englesbe et al,[17] 2010	163	50	Total psoas area had significant ($P < .0001$) effect on mortality after liver transplant with an adjusted HR = 0.27 (95% CI: 0.14–0.53) per 1000 mm² increase in psoas area
Figueiredo et al,[88] 2000	53	9.4–39.6	Comparing survivors and nonsurvivors, patients with longer ICU stay had lower HG on right (27 ± 6 and 36 ± 12 kg, $P = .01$) and left (27 ± 7 and 35 ± 12 kg, $P = .01$); lower lean body mass (51 ± 11 and 59 ± 14 kg, $P = .05$) 43% of patients experienced 1 or more episode of biopsy-proven acute cellular rejection and had significantly lower BMI (26 ± 6 and 29 ± 5 kg/m2, $P = .04$) and lower total body fat (21 ± 8 and 30 ± 9 kg, $P < .001$)

Le Cornu et al,[89] 2000	82	53	Malnutrition defined as MAMC <25th percentile, pretransplant nutritional status was not associated with survival; however, median survival in the group supplemented with calorie-dense enteral feed vs control had 90% vs 50% 1-y survival
Merli et al,[10] 2010	38	53	Estimated survival rate was 82.7% at 1 y, 65.1% at 3 y, and 50.7% at 5 y; MAMC <fifth percentile increased mortality risk based on relative risk = 1.79
Montano-Loza et al,[16] 2011	112	40	Only independent associations with mortality using multivariate Cox analysis were Child-Pugh (HR: 1.85; $P = .04$), MELD scores (HR: 1.08; $P = .001$), and sarcopenia (HR: 2.21; $P = .008$; Median survival time for patients with sarcopenia was 19 ± 6 mo compared with 34 ± 11 mo among patients without sarcopenic ($P = .005$)
Muller et al,[90] 1992	123	31	Posttransplantation mortality was independent of pretransplantation REE, but it increased significantly in patients with losses in BCM
Selberg et al,[5] 1997	150	46	Hypermetabolism as defined by ΔREE >20% and malnutrition defined by BCM <35% are present in significant proportion of patients awaiting liver transplant ($20.4 \pm 10\%$ and $33.8 \pm 6\%$).
Shahid et al,[91] 2005	61	30	MAC and TSF were significantly associated with postoperative death ($P = .04$ and $P = .02$); No statistically significant correlation between the nutritional measures and probability of acute rejection

Abbreviations: CI, confidence interval; HG, handgrip strength; HR, hazard ratio; ICU, intensive care unit; LOS, length of stay; LR, liver resection; LT, liver transplant; MAMC, midarm muscle circumference; MELD, model of end-stage liver disease; OR, odds ratio; PCM, protein calorie malnutrition; PNI, prognostic nutritional index; REE, resting energy expenditure; TSF, triceps skinfold thickness.

Summary: The impact of malnutrition on survival in cirrhosis is described in these 13 studies (n = 1187). The prevalence of pretransplant malnutrition was between 9.4% and 69.0%. Malnutrition is defined by BIA, HG, TSF, SGA, and total psoas area. The presence of malnutrition increased morbidity and mortality, including acute rejection after transplant and prolonged ICU stay. There is a statistically significant correlation between the severity of malnutrition and mortality.

and malnutrition worsen survival in cirrhosis, no studies have documented improved survival with reversal of sarcopenia. In this context, it is interesting that the authors' studies on reversal of sarcopenia after transjugular intrahepatic portosystemic shunt (TIPS) have demonstrated better survival after TIPS in patients in whom skeletal muscle mass increased compared with those in whom skeletal muscle mass did not change or became less.[92]

Malnutrition and Quality of Life

Quality of life in cirrhosis is significantly lower than that in controls (**Table 3**).[6,93–98] This finding has been related to the severity of underlying liver disease as assessed by the Child's scoring system. Because the Child's score relates to the severity and prevalence of malnutrition, it is expected that malnutrition will be related to the quality of life. Recently, in a prospective study of 61 patients with cirrhosis, those with malnutrition as defined by SGA had impairment in 6 of the 8 quality-of-life scales on the SF-36.[94] However, in patients with hepatocellular carcinoma, quality of life was not related to tumor mass or hepatocellular failure.[95] Similarly in patients with primary biliary cirrhosis, a condition with the most severe reduction in fat and muscle mass, the Nottingham health profile, a measure of quality of life, was not related to severity or duration of the disease.[96] However, in neither of these studies was the relation between malnutrition and quality of life evaluated. In summary, based on existing data, patients with cirrhosis and malnutrition as assessed by SGA had a worse quality of life than those with preserved muscle and fat mass. These findings were independent of the complications of cirrhosis. More recently, previous episodes of HE, even after complete resolution, impact the quality of life in patients with cirrhosis.[99] However, in a prospective study, minimal HE did not seem to have a significant impact on quality of life in patients with cirrhosis.[98] This finding was in contrast to clinical expectations and recent interest on the impact of minimal HE on driving skills and motor vehicle–related accidents.[100,101]

Malnutrition and Clinical Complications of Cirrhosis

The known major life-threatening complications of cirrhosis that include ascites, spontaneous bacterial peritonitis, portal hypertension and gastrointestinal bleeding, HE and hepatorenal syndrome, and all of these are adversely affected by malnutrition and sarcopenia (**Table 4**).[4,8,9,81,102–104] Other complications include hepatocellular carcinoma and pulmonary and cardiac complications of cirrhosis.[105] Each of these complications aggravates the catabolic state by their impact on circulating cytokines and hormones and results in the reduction of muscle mass.[35] However, few studies have systematically evaluated the impact of malnutrition on the development and progression of these complications. In a classical study by Moller,[106] the development of portal hypertension, portosystemic collaterals, and varices were more severe and common in malnourished patients. In this study, nutritional status was scored by a subjective assessment scale of 1 to 4, with 4 being cachexia. Even though the investigators do not describe the validation process of this scoring system, this study demonstrates that malnourished patients had more severe portal hypertension and risk of variceal bleeding.

In states of hepatocellular dysfunction and portal hypertension, plasma concentration of ammonia is elevated, and the skeletal muscle has been suggested to play a significant role in ammonia detoxification.[42,107] Because hyperammonemia is considered to be the major pathogenic factor in the development of HE, it has been speculated that low muscle mass will predispose to and aggravate the severity of HE. There are 2 studies that have specifically examined the impact of malnutrition on the development and outcome of HE with conflicting results.[7,108,109]

Both of these are single time-point cross-sectional assessments for malnutrition as defined by anthropometric and other criteria. In the study by Kalaitzakis and colleagues[7] in 128 patients with cirrhosis of varied causes, HE was diagnosed as overt by West Haven criteria and the number connection test. Malnutrition was defined by anthropometric measurement less than the fifth percentile of established norms for the general population, body mass index less than 20 mg/m^2, or weight loss of greater than or equal to 5% to 10% in the previous 3 to 6 months. Among these patients, 40% had malnutrition and 34% had HE. Patients with malnutrition had HE more frequently, and malnutrition was an independent risk factor for HE. In contrast, in another prospective study by Soros and colleagues,[108] nutritional assessment was performed using body mass index, anthropometrics using the triceps skinfold thickness and arm muscle area, and bioelectrical impedance. It is interesting that the 2 studies yielded conflicting results in terms of the impact of malnutrition on the development of HE. Unfortunately, both were cross-sectional studies and did not specifically examine the impact of sarcopenia on the development of HE. One of the major confounding factors in these assessments is that previous episodes of HE are also likely to worsen sarcopenia by a combination of hyperammonemia, poor oral intake, and hospitalizations. In a prospective study, the authors demonstrated that the frequency of HE was higher in patients who had evidence of sarcopenia.[110] The authors' studies in an animal model of hyperammonemia (portacaval anastomosis [PCA] rat) and in murine myoblasts have suggested that ammonia induces the expression of myostatin, a transforming growth factor (TGF) β superfamily member that is known to worsen sarcopenia.[111,112] The authors' data suggest that hyperammonemia of cirrhosis induces HE and worsens sarcopenia. The development and progression of sarcopenia then begins a self-destructive cycle of recurrent HE and further loss of muscle mass caused by impaired nonhepatic ammonia disposal.

PATHOGENESIS AND MECHANISMS OF SARCOPENIA IN CIRRHOSIS

Because sarcopenia is the major contributor to malnutrition, functional status, and outcomes in cirrhosis, an understanding of the biochemical and cellular mechanisms that result in loss of muscle mass is critical to identify therapeutic targets. Initial works in understanding the metabolic alterations in cirrhosis were based on isotopic tracer methodology.[113] Despite initial enthusiasm, these were predominantly descriptive studies; and only recently, the advances in myology, gerontology, and molecular biology are being translated into identifying precise molecular abnormalities in the skeletal muscle and their dysregulation in cirrhosis.[15,114]

Maintenance of Skeletal Muscle Mass

To understand the mechanisms of sarcopenia, an understanding of the mechanisms of maintenance of muscle mass is necessary (**Fig. 1**). Skeletal muscle mass is maintained by a balance between muscle protein synthesis, protein breakdown, and satellite cell proliferation and differentiation.[115] Satellite cells are myogenically committed precursor cells that contribute nuclei to the myocytes for maintenance and growth of mature skeletal muscle.[116,117] Increase in skeletal muscle protein synthesis and satellite cell proliferation and differentiation are necessary for skeletal muscle growth.[115] Satellite cells constitute 2% to 4% of adult skeletal muscle, whereas skeletal muscle structural protein is the major contributor to skeletal muscle mass. Therefore, alterations in skeletal muscle mass are primarily caused by changes in the structural protein content. Another critical concept that needs to be reiterated is that even though both impaired protein synthesis and increased protein breakdown

Table 3
Impact of malnutrition on quality of life in cirrhosis

Author/Year	n	Definition of Malnutrition	Prevalence of Malnutrition (%)	Quality-of-life Measures
Arguedas et al,[97] 2003	160	Not assessed	Not assessed	Patients completed the SF-36, those with advanced cirrhosis Child-Pugh class B/C, had significantly lower PCS scores compared with patients with Child-Pugh class A cirrhosis ($P = .02$); Patients with overt HE (grade I) had lower PCS scores compared with patients without HE ($P = .018$)
Kalaitzakis et al,[6] 2006	128	TSF, MAMC <10th percentile or BMI <20 kg m^2	19 in non EtOH cirrhosis, 53 in EtOH cirrhosis	Controls vs patients with cirrhosis showed higher gastrointestinal symptom severity (total GSRS score: 1.53, 95% CI: 1.50–1.55 vs 2.21, 95% CI: 2.04–2.38) and profound reductions in the SF-36 physical (47.0 95% CI: 45–49 vs 37.9 95% CI: 35.7–40.1) and mental component summary scores (51.0 95% CI: 49.0–53.0 vs 39.2 95% CI: 36.7–41.6)
Les et al,[93] 2010	212	BMI MAMC HG	Not assessed	HRQOL scores (global CLDQ = 4.8 ± 1.17, PCS = 38.6 ± 10.7, MCS = 45.3 ± 14.3) showed a decrease with worsening of liver function; There is a significant correlation between the Child-Pugh classification and the different domains of the CLDQ and the SF-36
Norman et al,[94] 2006	200	SGA A = well nourished SGA B, C = malnourished Anthropometric Handgrip strength	48	Malnourished vs well-nourished patients had decreased BMI (25.7 ± 4.6 vs 21.6 ± 4.2 kg/m^2), decreased BCM/height (8.6 ± 1.7 vs 7.4 ± 1.8 kg/m^2), decreased arm muscle area (4713.2 ± 1261.8 vs 3918 ± 1200.1) $P<.000$, decreased quality of life on chronic liver disease questionnaire, increased bodily pain (30% vs 40% $P<.01$), decreased social functioning 100% vs 70% $P<.01$), decreased mental health (70% vs 60% $P<.01$)

Poon et al,[95] 2004	41	Branched chain amino acid level	59	Patients with malnourished liver/ cirrhosis vs controls had decreased quality of life on FACT-G score 87 (65–98) vs 86 (74–99) at pretreatment and 89 (68–96) vs and 84 (70–96) P<.05; Patients transplanted for ALF or CLD had significantly worse HRQOL than the general population
Poupon et al,[96] 2004	276	Not assessed	Not assessed	Using the NHP to assess HRQOL, Patients with PBC showed a strong statistically significant difference in energy compared with controls (respectively, 40.6 vs 22.9, P<.0001) and had worse scores for emotional reactions (22.2 vs 16.1, P<.005)
Wunsch et al,[98] 2011	87	Not assessed	Not assessed	HRQOL was analyzed in patients without (n = 48) and patients with minimal HE (n = 29); Comparison of patients with vs without minimal HE, no differences in any of CLDQ and SF-36 domains

Abbreviations: ALF, acute liver failure; BCM, body cell mass; BMI, body mass index; CI, confidence interval; CLD, chronic liver disease; CLQD, chronic liver disease questionnaire; FACT-G, functional assessment of cancer therapy-general; GSRS, gastrointestinal symptoms severity score; HRQOL, health related quality of life; MAMC, midarm muscle circumference; NHP, Nottingham health profile; PBC, primary biliary cirrhosis; TSF, triceps skinfold thickness.

Summary: The impact of malnutrition on quality of life in cirrhosis is described in the previous 7 studies (n = 1104). Malnutrition is defined by BIA, MAMC, TSF, SGA, and branched chain amino acids levels. The prevalence of malnutrition ranged from 19% to 59%. Malnourished patients had statistically significant increase in gastrointestinal symptoms and decreased quality of life on the CLQD, SF-36, and NHP questionnaire.

Table 4
Impact of malnutrition on complications of liver disease in cirrhosis

Author/Year	n	Definition of Malnutrition	Prevalence of Malnutrition (%)	Complications of Liver Disease
All complications Alvares-da-Silva and Reverbel da,[4] 2005	50	SGA PNI HG	28 19 63	65.5% of malnourished subjects vs 11.8% of well-nourished subjects developed uncontrolled ascites, HE, SBP, and hepatorenal syndrome when assessed by HG ($P = .001$); 33.3% of malnourished subjects developed these major complications vs 46.2% well-nourished subjects when assessed by PNI ($P>.05$); 35.7% of malnourished subjects developed these complications vs 44.4% well-nourished subjects when assessed by SGA ($P>.05$)
Huisman et al,[8] 2011	84	HG MAMC SGA BCM BMI	67 58 58 39 5	Malnourished patients vs well-nourished patients had (48% vs 18%, $P = .007$) complications at follow-up, new-onset ascites (27% vs 18%, $P = .365$), HE (29% vs 0%, $P = .00$), hepatorenal (13% vs 0%, $P = .051$), SBP (14% vs 0%, $P = .035$); In univariate analysis using logistic regression, malnutrition measured with HG (OR: 4.3; CI: 1.4–12.9), $P<.2$ when comparing patients with and without complications during follow-up
SBP Merli et al,[9] 2010	38	SGA MAMC	53	73% of malnourished patients assessed by SGA had 1 or more infections; Total number of infective episodes per patient was significantly higher in malnourished patients compared with patients with no malnutrition, $P<.000001$; Total number of days in the ICU was influenced only by malnutrition (SGA A-B, C) HR 0.18; $P = .0003$
Portal HTN Sam and Nguyen,[81] 2009	114,703	Clinical diagnosis	6.1	PCM was higher among patients with cirrhosis and PHTN compared with general medical inpatients (6.1% vs 1.9%, $P<.0001$; OR: 1.55, 95% CI: 1.4–1.7) In patients with cirrhosis and PHTN, significantly higher rates of malnutrition in patients with alcohol abuse compared with those without (7.6% vs 4.7%, $P<.0001$), greater prevalence of ascites (64.6% vs 47.9%, $P<.0001$), and hepatorenal syndrome (5.1% vs 2.8% $P<.0001$) but not HE (60.8% vs 59.7%, $P = .11$) among patients with malnutrition and cirrhosis with PHTN

Montomoli et al,[102] 2010	21	BIA	30	TIPS procedure lowered portal pressure before compared with after (6.0 ± 2.1 mm Hg vs 15.8 ± 4.8 mm Hg, P<.001). After TIPS, normal-weight patients had an increase in dry lean mass (from 10.9 ± 5.9 kg to 12.7 ± 5.6 kg, P = .031) and TBW (from 34.5 ± 7.6 L to 40.2 ± 10.8 L, P = .007)
HE Kalaitzakis et al,[7] 2007	128	Anthropometry, MAC <fifth percentile	40	Patients with vs without malnutrition had more frequent episodes of HE (46% vs 27%; P = .031); There was no difference in episodes of HE comparing alcohol cause of liver disease vs other cause (49% vs 37%, P = .202), severity of cirrhosis by CP score (2.5% vs 2.2%, P = .09) or by MELD (6% vs 5%, P = .275)
Ndraha et al,[104] 2011	34	Prealbumin level	50	Malnourished patients randomized into groups received LOLA (group A) vs without LOLA (group B); CFF value in group A (2.41 ± 1.6 Hz) compared with group B (0.67 ± 2.3 Hz) P = .016; Increased incidence of minimal HE in patients with low MAMC; Minimal HE with malnutrition can be improved by use of L-ornithine-L-aspartate
Ascites Campillo et al,[192] 2003	396	MAMC, BMI, TSF <5th or 10th percentile	39	Prevalence of severe malnutrition highest in TAP (39.1%); Comparing TAP vs NAP, MAMC <5th or 10th percentile (65.5% vs 51.0%) and TSF <5th or 10th percentile (49.4% vs 30.4%) with P<.0001; In multivariate analysis, patients with TSF <5th or 10th percentile were positively associated with tense ascites (OR: 2.833, CI 95: 1.603–5.014, P = .0004)

Abbreviations: BCM, body cell mass; BMI, body mass index; CI, confidence interval; CP, Child Pugh; HG, handgrip strength; LOLA, L-ornithine-L-aspartate; MAMC, midarm muscle circumference; MELD, model end-stage liver disease; NAP, nonascitic patients with cirrhosis; OR, odds ratio; PCM, protein calorie malnutrition; PHTN, portal hypertension; PNI, prognostic nutritional index; SBP, spontaneous bacterial peritonitis; TAP, patients with cirrhosis with tense ascites; TBW, total body water; TSF, triceps skinfold.

Summary: Seven studies (n = 751) describe the impact of malnutrition on the complications of liver disease. Malnutrition is defined by BMI, HG, MAMC, TSF, and SGA. Prevalence of malnutrition is 6.1% to 67.0%. Complications of liver disease included are ascites, SBP, portal hypertension, hepatorenal syndrome, and HE. There is a statistically significant increase in complications in patients with malnutrition.

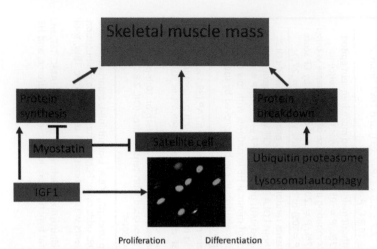

Proliferation   Differentiation

Fig. 1. Regulation of skeletal muscle mass. The protein synthesis and satellite cell (myogenically committed stem cells) contribute to muscle growth and reversal of atrophy. These are regulated primarily by myostatin and IGF1. The proteolysis is mediated primarily by the ubiquitin proteasome pathway with a variable contribution by the lysosomal cathepsin mediated autophagy pathway.

contribute to the reduced muscle mass in cirrhosis, their contributions are distinct. A reduction in protein synthesis alone results only in the failure to accrete protein mass, whereas an increase in proteolysis is necessary for the loss of muscle mass. However, continued enhanced proteolysis precludes cell survival and needs to be regulated. Because protein synthesis and proteolysis do not occur independently, rather are highly integrated, it is the relative contribution that determines the muscle mass. Current methods to quantify skeletal muscle protein synthesis and proteolysis lack sufficient sensitivity to identify the small changes that occur with the disease.[118] These methods are being supplemented by quantifying whole muscle protein synthesis instead of the traditional fractional synthesis rate in animal studies[36,119] but have not been developed in humans yet. Furthermore, there are no studies that have directly quantified skeletal muscle protein synthesis or breakdown in human cirrhosis. The use of isotopic tracers using stable isotope-labeled amino acids have examined whole body protein metabolism in cirrhosis.[1]

Protein Metabolism in Cirrhosis with Portosystemic Shunting

Protein turnover studies in cirrhosis using tracer isotopes have yielded conflicting results.[120–123] These differences may be related to confounding variables, such as differences in disease severity, nutritional status, and the methodology used to quantify protein turnover. The estimation of rates of whole body protein breakdown using [1-^{13}C]leucine, in humans with stable cirrhosis (defined as Child's class A or B) in the fasted state, were not different from those in healthy controls.[120] Studies using phenylalanine tracer showed a decreased whole body protein breakdown in patients with cirrhosis of Child's class B and C (decompensated) and no difference between compensated patients with cirrhosis (Child's class A and B) and healthy controls.[124,125] Contradictory results have been reported using different isotopic tracers, such as [^{15}N] glycine and [^{14}C] tyrosine.[126]

Several methods have been used to examine protein synthesis in vivo.[127] However, muscle biopsies are required for precise quantification of skeletal muscle protein synthesis. Even though these have not been reported in human patients with cirrhosis, whole body amino acid kinetic studies showed lower rates of protein synthesis in patients with cirrhosis than in controls.[121,123] Arteriovenous differences in amino acid concentration in the lower extremity showed that proteolysis and protein synthesis were lower.[123] These abnormalities may persist or worsen in the postprandial state in patients with cirrhosis.[121]

Data from studies in animal models are equally conflicting. In the rat model of carbon tetrachloride–induced cirrhosis, lower rate of protein breakdown and lower protein synthesis was observed.[128] In the PCA rat, a lower rate of liver and brain protein synthesis was reported 3 weeks after anastamosis.[129] In contrast, another study in PCA rats showed no difference in the rate of protein synthesis in different organs.[130] An increased skeletal muscle proteolysis mediated by the ubiquitin proteasome pathway has been described in the bile duct ligated rat.[131] However, the bile duct ligated rat as a model of cirrhosis differs from human cirrhosis because secondary biliary cirrhosis in humans is extremely rare and steatorrhea and malabsorption that accompany this procedure affect the muscle mass independent of cirrhosis.

Another pathway of protein breakdown that is being increasingly examined is the lysosomal cathepsin–mediated autophagy.[132,133] Autophagy serves to remove long-lived and abnormal proteins and dysfunctional organelles and helps recycle the substrates generated to permit protein synthesis. Autophagy is enhanced during states of nutrient deprivation and cellular stress. Preliminary studies from the authors' laboratory have shown an increased skeletal muscle autophagy. However, with the impaired muscle protein synthesis in cirrhosis, autophagy may be futile and contributes to sarcopenia, especially in the presence of reduced ubiquitin-proteasome–mediated proteolysis.

Despite the heterogeneity in the disease and methodologies used, the preponderance of evidence based on studies in humans and animals suggest an unchanged rate of protein breakdown and a decrease in the rate of protein synthesis in cirrhosis.[113,121,123] Several confounding variables may have contributed to the differences in observations and include the stage of the disease at the time of study, underlying cause of cirrhosis, duration of illness, muscle mass before disease development, and comorbid conditions that also contribute to whole body and skeletal muscle protein metabolism.

Satellite Cells and Skeletal Muscle Mass

Skeletal muscle fibers in adults are composed of terminally differentiated myocytes that do not replicate.[116,117] Their growth and adaptation to injury depend on a small population of stem cells called satellite cells that are committed to a myogenic lineage and are closely associated with the periphery of the muscle fibers.[117] Proliferation and differentiation of satellite cells contribute to the accretion of myonuclei in mature muscle cells and growth of skeletal muscle.[117,134] Impaired satellite cell proliferation and differentiation occur in sarcopenia of aging, calorie restriction, hind limb unloading, and immobilization.[135–137] However, the contribution of impaired satellite cell function to the diminished muscle mass in cirrhosis is unknown. The authors have shown in the PCA rat an impaired satellite cell proliferation and differentiation as evidenced by the low expression of proliferating cell nuclear antigen (PCNA) and myogenic regulatory factors (myoD, myf5, and myogenin).[38,39] The authors' in vivo immunohistochemical studies using 5 bromo 2' deoxyuridine incorporation have also shown that following PCA, there is a significantly lower mitotic index of satellitel cells compared with the control animals. These data suggest that satellite cell function is impaired in portosystemic shunting and may play a role in sarcopenia of cirrhosis. The enhancement of satellite cell function is a potential therapeutic target in these patients.

Molecular Regulation of Skeletal Muscle Protein Metabolism and Satellite Cell Function

There are 2 regulatory pathways that contribute to skeletal muscle growth: (1) enhanced protein synthesis in existing muscle fibers and (2) proliferation and differentiation of myogenic satellite cells that fuse with the exiting muscle fibers (**Fig. 2**). Myostatin and IGF1 are the 2 major upstream regulators of these functions in the skeletal muscle. An increase in skeletal muscle protein synthesis results from the activation of components of the highly regulated components of the canonical IGF1/PI3K/Akt/ mTOR signaling pathway (see **Fig. 1**).[115] Activation of Akt and mTOR by phosphorylation results in the stimulation of ribosomal protein translation by the effector proteins, p70s6k and 4E-BP.[138] The impairment of component proteins in this pathway results in reduced protein synthesis.[115,139] Proteolysis that is responsible for the reduction in muscle mass is also regulated by myostatin and IGF1. Impaired phosphorylation and activation of Akt results in increased ubiquitin proteasome–mediated proteolysis, and

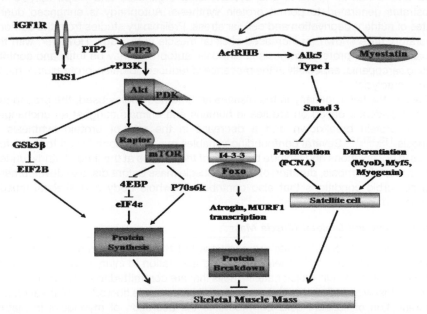

Fig. 2. Integration of the 3 major pathways that regulate skeletal muscle mass. Myostatin and IGF1 regulate muscle growth via transcriptional and posttranslational regulation of myogenic genes. The ubiquitin proteasome pathway is responsible for proteolysis. All 3 pathways crosstalk at multiple levels, including Akt, mTOR, AMP kinase, and FOXO. PIP2, phosphatidyl inositor bisphosphate; PIP3, phosphatidylinositol 3 phosphate; IGF1R, IGF1 receptor; Alk5, activinlike kinase 5, forms a heterodimeric complex with generic TGFβ receptor for myostatin; Act IIbr, activin II b receptor; GSK, 3β glycogen synthase kinase; eIF, eukaryotic initiation factor; 4E BP1, 4 E binding protein 1; IRS 1, insulin receptor substrate that is downstream of both insulin and IGF1 receptor; MURf, muscle ring finger protein, final component in the ubiquitin proteasome pathway with atrogin; PCNA, proliferating cell nuclear antigen, a marker of satellite cell proliferation.

reduced mTOR activation results in enhanced autophagy.[34,140] These results demonstrate the complex crosstalk at different components between the critical regulators of muscle mass and their ultimate targets and functional consequences.

Myostatin, a member of the TGF β superfamily expressed in the skeletal muscle, is a potent inhibitor of muscle protein synthesis and satellite cell function.[141] The authors have shown that the PCA rat is an appropriate model to examine the mechanisms responsible for failure to increase lean body weight and gain skeletal muscle mass with portosystemic shunting in cirrhosis.[40,111] The authors have previously reported that an increased expression of myostatin occurred 2 weeks after PCA and accompanied the failure to gain skeletal muscle mass and impaired satellite cell function.[38,39] This finding was accompanied by an impaired skeletal muscle protein synthetic response and decreased phosphorylation of mTOR and its downstream targets, p70s6 kinase and 4 E binding protein 1.[139] Others have shown that myostatin blocks an upstream regulator or mTOR (ie, protein kinase B or Akt.)[142,143] The administration of follistatin reversed the myostatin-induced loss of lean body mass, skeletal muscle weight, and impaired phosphorylation of mTOR and p70s6k.[36] Myostatin has also been shown to activate the ubiquitin proteasome–mediated proteolysis and the lysosomal autophagy.[140,144]

IGF1

In addition to myostatin, IGF1 is the other major factor that regulates skeletal muscle protein metabolism.[34] There is some evidence that locally produced IGF1 in the skeletal muscle (mechano-growth factor) mediates these effects rather than the circulating.[145] IGF1 increases muscle mass by promoting protein synthesis, inhibiting protein breakdown, and increasing satellite cell proliferation and differentiation. The intracellular signaling pathways downstream of IGF1 binding to its receptor, IGF1 receptor α (IGF1R α) have been well characterized.[115] Increased skeletal muscle protein synthesis and satellite cell proliferation in response to IGF1 are mediated by the activating Akt and sequential phosphorylation and activation of its downstream targets.[146,147] These data suggest that Akt is the central mediator of critical components of the pathway of protein synthesis in the skeletal muscle.

There is intense interest in the regulation of skeletal muscle IGF1 and myostatin in liver disease. Identification of the binding sites of both androgen receptor and nuclear factor kB on the promoter region of myostatin also holds promise as effective therapeutic targets. Translation of these data from animal and in vitro cell culture studies to humans is essential.

AGING PATIENTS WITH CIRRHOSIS

As the global population ages, this contributes to the progressive worsening of sarcopenia. It is estimated that after the age of 50 years, approximately 1% of skeletal muscle loss occurs per year.[148,149] The impact and interaction of sarcopenia of aging and cirrhosis are not known. The adverse effects of both of these processes on muscle mass and function may be exponential, contributing to an urgent need to increase our understanding of the mechanisms and identification of therapies.

POSTTRANSPLANTED PATIENTS WITH CIRRHOSIS

Pretransplant malnutrition, specifically sarcopenia, adversely impacts the perioperative and immediate posttransplant outcomes (**Table 5**). Additionally, pretransplant sarcopenia is associated with worse outcomes after liver transplantation.[5,17] It is thought that liver transplantation is curative for cirrhosis. However, it must be reiterated that

Table 5
Impact of malnutrition on liver transplant outcomes in cirrhosis

Author/Year	n	Definition of Malnutrition	Prevalence of Malnutrition (%)	Liver-Transplant Outcomes
de Carvalho et al,[76] 2010	70	Anthropometry; BIA	69 pretransplant; 63 posttransplant	Pretransplant 44.3% of patients had mild PCM and 24.3% had moderate or severe PCM; Univariate analysis of all patients at 90 d showed cirrhotic vs noncirrhotic (53.6×100% malnourished, $X^2 = 8.5$, $P = .004$) as an important factor associated with PCM; PCM was significantly increased in patients with cirrhosis compared with patients without cirrhosis at 90 d based on pretransplant PCM score (OR: 53.4, CI: 1.9–1481.9, $P = .019$) and 1 y after transplant based on TSF (OR: 7.202, CI: 1.2–44.1, $P = .033$)
Englesbe et al,[17] 2010	163	TPA	50	TPA had a significant ($P<.0001$) effect on mortality after liver transplant with an adjusted HR = 0.27 (95% CI: 0.14–0.53) per 1000 mm^2 increase in psoas area; 1-y survival ranged from 49.7% for small TPA vs 87.0% with large TPA
Figueiredo et al,[88] 2000	53	Anthropometry SGA Handgrip strength BCM	9.4–39.6	Comparing survivors and nonsurvivors, patients with longer ICU stay had lower handgrip strength on right (27 ± 6 and 36 ± 12 kg, $P = .01$) and left (27 ± 7 and 35 ± 12 kg, $P = .01$); lower lean body mass (51 ± 11 and 59 ± 14 kg, $P = .05$) 43% of patients experienced 1 or more episode of biopsy-proven acute cellular rejection and had significantly lower BMI (26 ± 6 and 29 ± 5 kg/m^2, $P = .04$) and lower total body fat (21 ± 8 and 30 ± 9 kg, $P<.001$)
Harrison et al,[190] 1997	102	MAMC <25th percentile TSF	28	Malnourished patients defined by MAMC <25th percentile have increased risk of infection compared with controls (66% vs 52%), increased susceptibility, decreased graft function (2 malnourished patients had primary nonfunction of their hepatic allograft); Malnourished patients had statistically significant difference in 6-mo postoperative mortality but not statistically significant (Wilcoxon-Gehan statistic, 199, $P = .09$); In multiple regression analysis with percentile position for MAMC as the dependent variable, significant relations were seen for age (beta = -0.15, T = -2.0, $P = .05$), and survival (beta = -0.18, T = -2.5, $P = .01$)

Study	n	Method	%	Findings
Merli et al,[10] 2010	38	Anthropometry, SGA	53	Pretransplant nutritional status was associated with number of episodes of infections and length of stay in ICU because 73% of malnourished patients assessed by SGA had 1 or more infections; Total number of infective episodes per patient was significantly higher in malnourished patients compared with patients with no malnutrition (85 vs 11) P<.000001; Total number of days in the ICU was influenced only be malnutrition (SGA A-B, C) HR: 0.18; P = .0003
Pikul et al,[56] 1994	69	SGA	79	Patients were categorized by SGA: 19% mild, 34% moderate, and 26% severely malnourished; Significant increase in number of days requiring ventilator support comparing mild vs severe (8 ± 10 vs 41 ± 37 d), hospital days (33 ± 13 vs 82 ± 40 d), and higher incidence of tracheostomy (15% vs 67%)
Selberg et al,[5] 1997	150	Anthropometry, BCM <35% BIA	50	Hypermetabolism as defined by ΔREE >20% and malnutrition defined by BCM <35% are present in significant proportion of patients awaiting liver transplant (20.4 ± 10% and 33.8 ± 6%) and correlate with survival after transplant; Comparing survival in patients with hypermetabolism and malnutrition vs controls is 60% vs 90%
Stephenson et al,[191] 2001	109	SGA	32–35	Using nutritional status as a lone preoperative variable using the Wilcoxon rank sum test, patients with severe malnutrition required more blood products intraoperatively comparing severely malnourished vs moderate (5.5 ± 5.5 vs 3.0 ± 6, P = .026; vs mild 1.5 ± 3, P<.0001); These patients had longer hospital stay, severe vs moderate (16 ± 9 vs 10 ± 5 d, P = .0027; vs mild 9 ± 8 d, P = .0006) First study to show that malnutrition was independent predictor of intraoperative transfusion requirements during OLT independent of UNOS status

Abbreviations: BCM, body cell mass; BIA, bioelectric impedance; BMI, body mass index; CI, confidence interval; HR, hazard ratio; ICU, intensive care unit; MAMC, midarm muscle circumference; OLT, orthotopic liver transplant; PCM, protein calorie malnutrition; REE, resting energy expenditure; TPA, total psoas area; TSF, triceps skinfold; UNOS, united network of organ sharing.

Summary: Eight studies (n = 754) assessed the impact of malnutrition on liver-transplant outcomes. Prevalence of malnutrition ranged form 9.4% to 79%. Malnutrition was defined by BIA, HG, MAMC, TSF, and SGA. Severe malnutrition independently predicted intraoperative complications, increased episodes of infection, increased length of stay in the ICU, acute cellular rejection, and increased transfusion requirements.

this option is available only to a minority of patients. Furthermore, posttransplant metabolic syndrome and the attendant insulin resistance adds to the worsening of muscle loss.[150,151] Finally, mTOR inhibitors, calcineurin inhibitors, and corticosteroids, commonly used immunosuppressants used after transplantation, alter the expression and activity of critical regulators of muscle protein metabolism.[152–154] These observations support the urgent need to develop therapies to reverse and treat sarcopenia in cirrhosis because this casts a long shadow from before transplantation to after the procedure.

THERAPEUTIC OPTIONS

Given the human data that suggest that cirrhosis is a state of accelerated starvation,[155] several nutrient interventions have been tried with limited success in long-term improvement in protein or energy metabolism.[156,157] Several hormonal alterations have resulted in interventions that use anabolic androgens, IGF, and growth hormone with no benefit and several adverse effects.[158–161] Current studies underway on understanding the mechanisms of alteration in protein and fat malnutrition in cirrhosis are likely to provide the basis of novel treatment options (**Table 6**). Methods to determine the nutritional needs have also been devised and include quantification of the resting energy expenditure (REE), respiratory quotient (RQ), and daily protein needs.

The standard method to measure REE and RQ is the use of a metabolic cart. However, cost, logistics, and complexity of the test have led to this being used only in research settings. Interest has increased recently in the use of a handheld calorimeter that has been found to be more precise than a variety of predictive equations. In hospitalized patients with cirrhosis, the authors have found the handheld respiratory calorimeter (MedGem, Microlife Medical Home Solutions, Inc., CO, USA) to be as precise as a metabolic cart in the clinical research unit in quantifying REE. The European Society for Clinical Nutrition and Metabolism guidelines suggest no protein restriction in patients with cirrhosis based on published studies.[157]

NUTRITIONAL SUPPLEMENTATION

Because skeletal muscle is the major whole body protein store, with a reduction in muscle mass, whole body protein content is lower. Increased protein intake has been demonstrated to be safe, well tolerated, and beneficial in patients with cirrhosis, but the long-term anabolic effects on muscle mass and function have not yet been established.[33,156,162–166] Several nutritional interventions have been examined that have focused on 2 specific areas: decrease the intermeal frequency and increase caloric and protein intake (**Table 7**).[93,103,167–171] However, as stated earlier, recent advances in our understanding of skeletal muscle biology, regulatory pathways, and targeted interventions have not been evaluated. Separation of adipocyte and skeletal muscle responses to specific interventions are likely to result in the reversal of sarcopenia without the accompanying increase in fat mass and to avoid the development of sarcopenic obesity.

Dietary modification and supplements have been examined with conflicting results. Frequent snacks, late-evening snacks, branched chain amino acid supplementation, breakfast, and protein supplementation have been examined with beneficial results but have not been incorporated into routine clinical practice.[22,171–173] There is increasing evidence that shortening the interval between meals will reduce the severity and prevalence of malnutrition in cirrhosis.[22] Hence, the emphasis has been on late-evening snacks and, recently, on breakfast on waking up.[22,171] Both these measures have the benefit of increasing the availability of amino acids and suppressing gluconeogenesis from amino acids derived from endogenous proteolysis. Furthermore, both splanchnic and whole body protein breakdown are suppressed by dietary intake. Late-evening snacks have been shown to improve whole body protein kinetics with lower protein breakdown and increased protein synthesis. However, these are short-term effects. Animal data in the portacaval shunted rat model suggest that early in the course of the illness, there is increased proteolysis; and later, once loss of muscle and fat mass is established, there is an impaired skeletal muscle protein synthesis.[39] This interpretation is supported by studies in stable patients with cirrhosis in whom there is increased whole body protein breakdown.[33] The stage of the disease and underlying cause affect the severity of malnutrition in humans. However, the authors' animal data suggest that the duration of illness plays a significant role, with increased proteolysis early and impaired protein synthesis late in the disease.[36] Therefore, the therapeutic strategy will be to focus on reducing muscle proteolysis early in the disease and promote muscle protein synthesis later in the disease once muscle loss is established. Furthermore, the authors' observation of increased skeletal muscle autophagy is novel and needs further studies for its implications in the pathogenesis and reversal of sarcopenia in cirrhosis.

Of the essential amino acids, leucine holds the most promise as an intervention to reverse sarcopenia in aging.[174,175] Leucine is not only an essential amino acid substrate for protein synthesis but also functions as a direct activator of the critical protein synthesis and autophagy regulator, mTOR.[176] Additionally, leucine stimulates insulin release from the pancreatic β cells that functions as an anabolic hormone in the skeletal muscle.[177] Finally, leucine is an energy substrate in the skeletal muscle. However, because the administration of leucine will stimulate muscle protein synthesis, other essential amino acids may become limiting and need to be replaced.[178] Leucine-enriched essential amino acids can, therefore, be considered in the long-term management of sarcopenia of cirrhosis. It has been identified that reversing sarcopenia and cachexia can improve outcome in other disorders, like cancer.[179] A similar therapeutic approach in patients with cirrhosis is likely to improve survival, quality of life, and the development of other complications. Such outcome measures have not yet been reported. The authors recently showed that in response to TIPS, a subgroup of patients had an improvement in muscle size measured on CT. These patients had significantly better survival compared with those who either did not increase or had a reduction in muscle size.[92]

Micronutrient Replacement

Even though the authors have not focused on micronutrient replacement in cirrhosis, deficiency of vitamin D and zinc are well recognized and need to be identified and treated.[180–184]

Exercise

The role of aerobic and resistance exercise on skeletal muscle insulin signaling, protein synthesis response, AMP kinase activity, and satellite cell function has been studied extensively in aging.[185,186] However, fatigue; reduced maximum exercise capacity in patients with cirrhosis; and the presence of limiting complications, including ascites, encephalopathy, and portal hypertension, have limited the translation of the data or the elegant designs of the studies performed in patients without cirrhosis.[187] Resistance exercise increases portal hypertension, and even transient increases in portal hypertension can result in catastrophic variceal bleeding and

Table 6
Therapeutic options for malnutrition in cirrhosis

Author/Year	n	Definition of Malnutrition	Prevalence of Malnutrition (%)	Therapeutic Intervention	Response
Campillo et al,[103] 1997	55	MAMC <fifth percentile TSF <25th percentile	73 51	Oral nutrition	Patients with cirrhosis were given oral nutrition with caloric intake of ~40 kcal/kg of BW, this study compared Child A, B, C classification. FM increased from 17.4% ± 1.7%–19.5% ± 1.4%, $P<.01$, in Child A patients; from 17.1% ± 1.4%–19.3% ± 1.4%, $P<.001$, in Child B patients; and from 17.6% ± 1.5%–18.8% ± 1.5%, $P<.05$, in Child C patients, all categories received oral nutrition; Increase in FM was comparable in 3 groups, no significant increase in MAMC, TSF, or creatinine/height ratio
Kondrup et al,[165] 1997	11	BW <80% of reference weight, or LBM <80% of reference value LBM was calculated from three 24-h urinary creatinine excretions	57	Oral nutrition, high-protein diet	Patients were initially in energy balance (intake 7.9 ± 0.7) MJ per day vs energy expenditure (7.5 ± 0.3) MJ per day; During refeeding, energy intake was increased in proportion to protein intake; Malnourished patients with cirrhosis have both high protein use and require increased amount of protein to achieve nitrogen balance because of an increase in protein degradation; It is speculated that this is caused by low levels of IGF-I secondary to impaired liver function because initial plasma concentration of IGF-I was about 25% of control values and remained low during refeeding

Study	n	Assessment		Intervention	Results
Nielsen et al,[168] 1995	15	BW <80% of reference weight, or LBM <80% of reference value; LBM was calculated from three 24-h urinary creatinine excretions	63	Oral nutrition	Malnourished patients with EtOH cirrhosis were given increasing amounts of a balanced ordinary diet for 38 ± 3 d; Total nitrogen disposal was calculated after measurement of urinary and fecal nitrogen loss; Initial protein balance noted to be 0.50 ± 0.17 g/kg/d in malnourished patients with cirrhosis; Refeeding resulted in doubled protein intake from 0.98 ± 0.08 vs 1.78 ± 0.11 g/kg/d; increased anthropometric values, LBM (72-h creatinine) 2.4 ± 0.6 kg ($P<.005$); MAMA 3.1 ± 0.5 cm² ($P<.001$) and TSF 0.7 ± 0.3 mm ($P<.05$)
Plauth et al,[169] 2000	16	Serum ammonia and glutamine level	Not assessed	Enteral nutrition vs parenteral nutrition	Using TIPS to examine mesenteric venous blood, both glutamine and ammonia concentrations were measured in patients with cirrhosis; Patients that were given enteral nutrient infusion, ammonia release increased rapidly compared with postabsorptive state 65 (58–73) vs 107 (95–119) µmol/l after 15 min (95% CI) compared with parenteral infusion 50 (41–59) vs 62 (47–77) µmol/l; There was a higher blood ammonia: 14 (11–17) vs 9 (6–12) µmol/l in enteral compared with parenteral nutrition; These data indicate small intestinal metabolism contributes to hyperammonemia, therefore, parenteral nutrition is superior to enteral

(continued on next page)

Table 6
(continued)

Author/Year	n	Definition of Malnutrition	Prevalence of Malnutrition (%)	Therapeutic Intervention	Response
Swart et al,[170] 1989	8	BCAA level	50	Oral nutrition, 40-g protein diet	Comparing the effect of nitrogen balance on BCAA protein and natural protein, patients were in a negative nitrogen balance on a 40-g protein diet (-0.75 ± 0.15 gN) and in positive nitrogen balance on 60 g ($+1.23 \pm 0.22$ gN) or 80 g of protein per day ($+2.77 \pm 0.20$ gN); Patients with higher nitrogen balance had improved physical condition, mean minimum protein requirement (48 ± 5 g of protein per day or 0.75 g/kg/d), and decreased episodes of HE
Vaisman et al,[171] 2010	21	Serum ammonia level >85 μg/dl	Not assessed	Oral nutrition, 4–7 meals per day	Patients with cirrhosis with levels of ammonia >85 μg/dl scored significantly lower global cognitive score 92 ± 10.6 vs 100 ± 5.9 ($P<.015$) in healthy controls. PCM is prevalent in all clinical stages of liver disease. In patients with cirrhosis, attention (3.6 ± 10.6 vs 4.09 ± 2.93) and executive function (6.38 ± 9.06 vs -0.63 ± 4.11) increased with breakfast compared with without breakfast ($P = .04$)

Abbreviations: BCAA, branched chain amino acid; BW, body weight; EtOH cirrhosis, alcoholic cirrhosis; FM, fat mass; LBM, lean body mass; MAMA, midarm muscle area; MAMC, midarm muscle circumference; MJ, megajoule; PCM, protein calorie malnutrition; TSF, triceps skinfold.

Summary: Six studies (n = 126) describe the therapeutic interventions for malnutrition in cirrhosis. Malnutrition is defined by BCAA, BW, LBM, MAMC, serum ammonia and glutamine level, and TSF. Prevalence of malnutrition is 50% to 73% and was not assessed in 2 studies. Therapeutic options include modified eating patterns with increased protein through either oral nutrition or parenteral. Malnourished patients are noted to have increase in other complications of cirrhosis, including ascites, spontaneous bacterial peritonitis, portal hypertension, hepatorenal syndrome, and HE. There is a statistically significant increase in LBM and FM in patients with cirrhosis with improved oral or parenteral nutrition.

Table 7
Pathophysiology-based therapeutic options

Mechanism	Therapy	Response
Hyperammonemia	Lactulose, rifaximin	Not assessed
Low branched chain amino acids	Replace with BCAA	Partial response
Low leucine	Leucine-enriched essential amino acids	Not evaluated
Increased gluconeogenesis, accelerated starvation	Late-evening snack	Partially effective
Low IGF	IGF1, growth hormone	Not effective
Low androgens	Testosterone, oxandrolone	Partially effective
Increased myostatin	Myostatin antagonists	Not studied
Decreased physical activity	Aerobic and resistance exercise	Not effective, risk of variceal bleeding
Portal hypertension	TIPS	Improves muscle size and lean body mass

Abbreviation: BCAA, branched chain amino acid.

death.[188] It is, therefore, critical that the data on the impact of exercise on muscle mass and function be translated very judiciously in patients with cirrhosis.

Novel strategies to reverse cachexia, including myostatin antagonists, are also of clinical interest, especially given recent data that myostatin may play a critical role in cirrhotic sarcopenia.[35,189] The authors' data in an animal model that the adverse consequences of increased myostatin expression can be reversed without impacting the underlying liver disease are especially exciting[36] because liver transplantation is not a universally available treatment option and reversing hepatic cachexia-sarcopenia should be a major therapeutic option for cirrhosis. Given the paucity of data, the understudied nature of the problem, sarcopenia in cirrhosis deserves to be recognized as an area of unmet need with the potential to improve the outcome of the large number of patients with cirrhosis. One potential strategy for the development of novel and successful therapies is the need for consilience between the diverse and seemingly unrelated fields of aging, molecular signaling, nutraceuticals, hepatology, transplant immunology, clinical nutrition, and transplant surgeons.

REFERENCES

1. Tessari P. Protein metabolism in liver cirrhosis: from albumin to muscle myofibrils. Curr Opin Clin Nutr Metab Care 2003;6(1):79–85.
2. Bianchi G, Marzocchi R, Agostini F, et al. Update on nutritional supplementation with branched-chain amino acids. Curr Opin Clin Nutr Metab Care 2005;8(1): 83–7.
3. Bilbao I, Armadans L, Lazaro JL, et al. Predictive factors for early mortality following liver transplantation. Clin Transplant 2003;17(5):401–11.
4. Alvares-da-Silva MR, Reverbel da ST. Comparison between handgrip strength, subjective global assessment, and prognostic nutritional index in assessing malnutrition and predicting clinical outcome in cirrhotic outpatients. Nutrition 2005;21(2):113–7.

5. Selberg O, Bottcher J, Tusch G, et al. Identification of high- and low-risk patients before liver transplantation: a prospective cohort study of nutritional and metabolic parameters in 150 patients. Hepatology 1997;25(3):652–7.

6. Kalaitzakis E, Simren M, Olsson R, et al. Gastrointestinal symptoms in patients with liver cirrhosis: associations with nutritional status and health-related quality of life. Scand J Gastroenterol 2006;41(12):1464–72.

7. Kalaitzakis E, Olsson R, Henfridsson P, et al. Malnutrition and diabetes mellitus are related to hepatic encephalopathy in patients with liver cirrhosis. Liver Int 2007;27(9):1194–201.

8. Huisman EJ, Trip EJ, Siersema PD, et al. Protein energy malnutrition predicts complications in liver cirrhosis. Eur J Gastroenterol Hepatol 2011;23(11):982–9.

9. Merli M, Lucidi C, Giannelli V, et al. Cirrhotic patients are at risk for health care-associated bacterial infections. Clin Gastroenterol Hepatol 2010;8(11):979–85.

10. Merli M, Giusto M, Gentili F, et al. Nutritional status: its influence on the outcome of patients undergoing liver transplantation. Liver Int 2010;30(2):208–14.

11. O'Brien A, Williams R. Nutrition in end-stage liver disease: principles and practice. Gastroenterology 2008;134(6):1729–40.

12. Kerwin AJ, Nussbaum MS. Adjuvant nutrition management of patients with liver failure, including transplant. Surg Clin North Am 2011;91(3):565–78.

13. Ferreira LG, Anastacio LR, Correia MI. The impact of nutrition on cirrhotic patients awaiting liver transplantation. Curr Opin Clin Nutr Metab Care 2010; 13(5):554–61.

14. Argiles JM, Anker SD, Evans WJ, et al. Consensus on cachexia definitions. J Am Med Dir Assoc 2010;11(4):229–30.

15. Evans WJ, Morley JE, Argiles J, et al. Cachexia: a new definition. Clin Nutr 2008; 27(6):793–9.

16. Montano-Loza AJ, Meza-Junco J, Prado CM, et al. Sarcopenia is associated with mortality in patients with cirrhosis. Clin Gastroenterol Hepatol 2011. [Epub ahead of print].

17. Englesbe MJ, Patel SP, He K, et al. Sarcopenia and mortality after liver transplantation. J Am Coll Surg 2010;211(2):271–8.

18. Peng S, Plank LD, McCall JL, et al. Body composition, muscle function, and energy expenditure in patients with liver cirrhosis: a comprehensive study. Am J Clin Nutr 2007;85(5):1257–66.

19. Alberino F, Gatta A, Amodio P, et al. Nutrition and survival in patients with liver cirrhosis. Nutrition 2001;17(6):445–50.

20. Campillo B, Richardet JP, Bories PN. Enteral nutrition in severely malnourished and anorectic cirrhotic patients in clinical practice. Gastroenterol Clin Biol 2005; 29(6–7):645–51.

21. Plauth M, Schutz ET. Cachexia in liver cirrhosis. Int J Cardiol 2002;85(1):83–7.

22. Tsien CD, McCullough AJ, Dasarathy S. Late evening snack - exploiting a period of anabolic opportunity in cirrhosis. J Gastroenterol Hepatol 2011. [Epub ahead of print].

23. Nutritional status in cirrhosis. Italian multicentre cooperative project on nutrition in liver cirrhosis. J Hepatol 1994;21(3):317–25.

24. Lata J, Husova L, Jurankova J, et al. Factors participating in the development and mortality of variceal bleeding in portal hypertension–possible effects of the kidney damage and malnutrition. Hepatogastroenterology 2006;53(69): 420–5.

25. Gunsar F, Raimondo ML, Jones S, et al. Nutritional status and prognosis in cirrhotic patients. Aliment Pharmacol Ther 2006;24(4):563–72.

26. Marchesini G, Marzocchi R, Noia M, et al. Branched-chain amino acid supplementation in patients with liver diseases. J Nutr 2005;135(Suppl 6):1596S–601S.

27. Kato M, Miwa Y, Tajika M, et al. Preferential use of branched-chain amino acids as an energy substrate in patients with liver cirrhosis. Intern Med 1998;37(5):429–34.

28. Tsiaousi ET, Hatzitolios AI, Trygonis SK, et al. Malnutrition in end stage liver disease: recommendations and nutritional support. J Gastroenterol Hepatol 2008;23(4):527–33.

29. Charlton M. Branched-chain amino acid enriched supplements as therapy for liver disease. J Nutr 2006;136(Suppl 1):295S–8S.

30. Conchillo M, de Knegt RJ, Payeras M, et al. Insulin-like growth factor I (IGF-I) replacement therapy increases albumin concentration in liver cirrhosis: results of a pilot randomized controlled clinical trial. J Hepatol 2005;43(4):630–6.

31. Zaratiegui M, Castilla-Cortazar I, Garcia M, et al. IGF1 gene transfer into skeletal muscle using recombinant adeno-associated virus in a rat model of liver cirrhosis. J Physiol Biochem 2002;58(3):169–76.

32. Bucuvalas JC, Horn JA, Chernausek SD. Resistance to growth hormone in children with chronic liver disease. Pediatr Transplant 1997;1(1):73–9.

33. Biolo G, Antonione R, Barazzoni R, et al. Mechanisms of altered protein turnover in chronic diseases: a review of human kinetic studies. Curr Opin Clin Nutr Metab Care 2003;6(1):55–63.

34. Glass D, Roubenoff R. Recent advances in the biology and therapy of muscle wasting. Ann N Y Acad Sci 2010;1211:25–36.

35. Ruegg MA, Glass DJ. Molecular mechanisms and treatment options for muscle wasting diseases. Annu Rev Pharmacol Toxicol 2011;51:373–95.

36. Dasarathy S, McCullough AJ, Muc S, et al. Sarcopenia associated with portosystemic shunting is reversed by follistatin. J Hepatol 2011;54(5):915–21.

37. Gayan-Ramirez G, van de Casteele M, Rollier H, et al. Biliary cirrhosis induces type IIx/b fiber atrophy in rat diaphragm and skeletal muscle, and decreases IGF-I mRNA in the liver but not in muscle. J Hepatol 1998;29(2):241–9.

38. Dasarathy S, Dodig M, Muc SM, et al. Skeletal muscle atrophy is associated with an increased expression of myostatin and impaired satellite cell function in the portacaval anastomosis rat. Am J Physiol Gastrointest Liver Physiol 2004; 287(6):G1124–30.

39. Dasarathy S, Muc S, Hisamuddin K, et al. Altered expression of genes regulating skeletal muscle mass in the portacaval anastomosis rat. Am J Physiol Gastrointest Liver Physiol 2007;292(4):G1105–13.

40. Dasarathy S, Mullen KD, Dodig M, et al. Inhibition of aromatase improves nutritional status following portacaval anastomosis in male rats. J Hepatol 2006; 45(2):214–20.

41. Canturk NZ, Canturk Z, Ozden M, et al. Protective effect of IGF-1 on experimental liver cirrhosis-induced common bile duct ligation. Hepatogastroenterology 2003;50(54):2061–6.

42. Holecek M, Kandar R, Sispera L, et al. Acute hyperammonemia activates branched-chain amino acid catabolism and decreases their extracellular concentrations: different sensitivity of red and white muscle. Amino Acids 2011;40(2):575–84.

43. Sriram S, Subramanian S, Sathiakumar D, et al. Modulation of reactive oxygen species in skeletal muscle by myostatin is mediated through NF-kappaB. Aging Cell 2011;10(6):931–48.

44. Chinn KS. Prediction of muscle and remaining tissue protein in man. J Appl Physiol 1967;23(5):713–5.

45. Krzywicki HJ, Chinn KS. Body composition of a military population, Fort Carson, 1963. I. Body density, fat, and potassium 40. Am J Clin Nutr 1967;20(7):708–15.
46. Krzywicki HJ, Chinn KS. Human body density and fat of an adult male population as measured by water displacement. Am J Clin Nutr 1967;20(4):305–10.
47. Krzywicki HJ, Chinn KS. Body composition of a military population, Fort Carson, 1963. I. Body density, fat and potassium 40. Lab Rep 296. Rep US Army Med Res Nutr Lab Denver 1966;22:1–17.
48. DiCecco SR, Wieners EJ, Wiesner RH, et al. Assessment of nutritional status of patients with end-stage liver disease undergoing liver transplantation. Mayo Clin Proc 1989;64(1):95–102.
49. Hasse J, Strong S, Gorman MA, et al. Subjective global assessment: alternative nutrition-assessment technique for liver-transplant candidates. Nutrition 1993; 9(4):339–43.
50. Hasse JM. Nutritional implications of liver transplantation. Henry Ford Hosp Med J 1990;38(4):235–40.
51. O'Keefe SJ, El-Zayadi AR, Carraher TE, et al. Malnutrition and immuno-incompetence in patients with liver disease. Lancet 1980;2(8195 pt 1):615–7.
52. Sobhonslidsuk A, Roongpisuthipong C, Nantiruj K, et al. Impact of liver cirrhosis on nutritional and immunological status. J Med Assoc Thai 2001;84(7):982–8.
53. Francoz C, Prie D, Abdelrazek W, et al. Inaccuracies of creatinine and creatinine-based equations in candidates for liver transplantation with low creatinine: impact on the model for end-stage liver disease score. Liver Transpl 2010; 16(10):1169–77.
54. Thuluvath PJ, Triger DR. How valid are our reference standards of nutrition? Nutrition 1995;11(6):731–3.
55. Thuluvath PJ, Triger DR. Evaluation of nutritional status by using anthropometry in adults with alcoholic and nonalcoholic liver disease. Am J Clin Nutr 1994; 60(2):269–73.
56. Pikul J, Sharpe MD, Lowndes R, et al. Degree of preoperative malnutrition is predictive of postoperative morbidity and mortality in liver transplant recipients. Transplantation 1994;57(3):469–72.
57. Fuller NJ, Jebb SA, Goldberg GR, et al. Inter-observer variability in the measurement of body composition. Eur J Clin Nutr 1991;45(1):43–9.
58. Godoy R, Goodman E, Levins R, et al. Anthropometric variability in the USA: 1971-2002. Ann Hum Biol 2005;32(4):469–86.
59. Akerman PA, Jenkins RL, Bistrian BR. Preoperative nutrition assessment in liver transplantation. Nutrition 1993;9(4):350–6.
60. Horber FF, Thomi F, Casez JP, et al. Impact of hydration status on body composition as measured by dual energy x-ray absorptiometry in normal volunteers and patients on haemodialysis. Br J Radiol 1992;65(778):895–900.
61. Pirlich M, Schutz T, Spachos T, et al. Bioelectrical impedance analysis is a useful bedside technique to assess malnutrition in cirrhotic patients with and without ascites. Hepatology 2000;32(6):1208–15.
62. Madden AM, Morgan MY. The potential role of dual-energy x-ray absorptiometry in the assessment of body composition in cirrhotic patients. Nutrition 1997; 13(1):40–5.
63. Morgan MY, Madden AM, Jennings G, et al. Two-component models are of limited value for the assessment of body composition in patients with cirrhosis. Am J Clin Nutr 2006;84(5):1151–62.
64. Chinn KS, Hannon JP. Relationship of muscle protein to other components of the fat-free mass. Am J Physiol 1966;211(4):993–7.

65. Morgan MY, Madden AM. The assessment of body composition in patients with cirrhosis. Eur J Nucl Med 1996;23(2):213–25.
66. Madden AM, Morgan MY. A comparison of skinfold anthropometry and bioelectrical impedance analysis for measuring percentage body fat in patients with cirrhosis. J Hepatol 1994;21(5):878–83.
67. Fuller NJ, Jebb SA, Laskey MA, et al. Four-component model for the assessment of body composition in humans: comparison with alternative methods, and evaluation of the density and hydration of fat-free mass. Clin Sci (Lond) 1992;82(6):687–93.
68. Mendenhall CL, Anderson S, Weesner RE, et al. Protein-calorie malnutrition associated with alcoholic hepatitis. Veterans Administration Cooperative Study Group on Alcoholic Hepatitis. Am J Med 1984;76(2):211–22.
69. Lautz HU, Selberg O, Korber J, et al. Protein-calorie malnutrition in liver cirrhosis. Clin Investig 1992;70(6):478–86.
70. Addolorato G, Capristo E, Greco AV, et al. Influence of chronic alcohol abuse on body weight and energy metabolism: is excess ethanol consumption a risk factor for obesity or malnutrition? J Intern Med 1998;244(5):387–95.
71. Caly WR, Strauss E, Carrilho FJ, et al. Different degrees of malnutrition and immunological alterations according to the aetiology of cirrhosis: a prospective and sequential study. Nutr J 2003;2:10.
72. Caregaro L, Alberino F, Amodio P, et al. Malnutrition in alcoholic and virus-related cirrhosis. Am J Clin Nutr 1996;63(4):602–9.
73. Roongpisuthipong C, Sobhonslidsuk A, Nantiruj K, et al. Nutritional assessment in various stages of liver cirrhosis. Nutrition 2001;17(9):761–5.
74. Figueiredo FA, De Mello PR, Kondo M. Effect of liver cirrhosis on body composition: evidence of significant depletion even in mild disease. J Gastroenterol Hepatol 2005;20(2):209–16.
75. Lehnert ME, Clarke DD, Gibbons JG, et al. Estimation of body water compartments in cirrhosis by multiple-frequency bioelectrical-impedance analysis. Nutrition 2001;17(1):31–4.
76. de Carvalho L, Parise ER, Samuel D. Factors associated with nutritional status in liver transplant patients who survived the first year after transplantation. J Gastroenterol Hepatol 2010;25(2):391–6.
77. Hehir DJ, Jenkins RL, Bistrian BR, et al. Nutrition in patients undergoing orthotopic liver transplant. JPEN J Parenter Enteral Nutr 1985;9(6):695–700.
78. Loguercio C, Sava E, Sicolo P, et al. Nutritional status and survival of patients with liver cirrhosis: anthropometric evaluation. Minerva Gastroenterol Dietol 1996;42(2):57–60.
79. Mills PR, Shenkin A, Anthony RS, et al. Assessment of nutritional status and in vivo immune responses in alcoholic liver disease. Am J Clin Nutr 1983;38(6):849–59.
80. Reisman Y, Gips CH, Lavelle SM. Assessment of liver cirrhosis severity in 1015 patients of the Euricterus database with Campbell-Child, Pugh-Child and with ascites and ascites-nutritional state (ANS) related classifications. Euricterus Project Management Group. Hepatogastroenterology 1997;44(17):1376–84.
81. Sam J, Nguyen GC. Protein-calorie malnutrition as a prognostic indicator of mortality among patients hospitalized with cirrhosis and portal hypertension. Liver Int 2009;29(9):1396–402.
82. Tai ML, Goh KL, Mohd-Taib SH, et al. Anthropometric, biochemical and clinical assessment of malnutrition in Malaysian patients with advanced cirrhosis. Nutr J 2010;9:27.

83. Rantanen T, Harris T, Leveille SG, et al. Muscle strength and body mass index as long-term predictors of mortality in initially healthy men. J Gerontol A Biol Sci Med Sci 2000;55(3):M168–73.

84. Durand F, Valla D. Assessment of the prognosis of cirrhosis: Child-Pugh versus MELD. J Hepatol 2005;42(Suppl 1):S100–7.

85. Figueiredo FA, Perez RM, Freitas MM, et al. Comparison of three methods of nutritional assessment in liver cirrhosis: subjective global assessment, traditional nutritional parameters, and body composition analysis. J Gastroenterol 2006;41(5):476–82.

86. Bathgate AJ, Hynd P, Sommerville D, et al. The prediction of acute cellular rejection in orthotopic liver transplantation. Liver Transpl Surg 1999;5(6):475–9.

87. Deschenes M, Villeneuve JP, Dagenais M, et al. Lack of relationship between preoperative measures of the severity of cirrhosis and short-term survival after liver transplantation. Liver Transpl Surg 1997;3(5):532–7.

88. Figueiredo F, Dickson ER, Pasha T, et al. Impact of nutritional status on outcomes after liver transplantation. Transplantation 2000;70(9):1347–52.

89. Le Cornu KA, McKiernan FJ, Kapadia SA, et al. A prospective randomized study of preoperative nutritional supplementation in patients awaiting elective orthotopic liver transplantation. Transplantation 2000;69(7):1364–9.

90. Muller MJ, Lautz HU, Plogmann B, et al. Energy expenditure and substrate oxidation in patients with cirrhosis: the impact of cause, clinical staging and nutritional state. Hepatology 1992;15(5):782–94.

91. Shahid M, Johnson J, Nightingale P, et al. Nutritional markers in liver allograft recipients. Transplantation 2005;79(3):359–62.

92. Tsien CD, Shah S, Runkana A, et al. Reversal of sarcopenia predicts survival after transjugular intrahepatic portosystemic stent. Hepatology 2011. [Epub ahead of print].

93. Les I, Doval E, Flavia M, et al. Quality of life in cirrhosis is related to potentially treatable factors. Eur J Gastroenterol Hepatol 2010;22(2):221–7.

94. Norman K, Kirchner H, Lochs H, et al. Malnutrition affects quality of life in gastroenterology patients. World J Gastroenterol 2006;12(21):3380–5.

95. Poon RT, Yu WC, Fan ST, et al. Long-term oral branched chain amino acids in patients undergoing chemoembolization for hepatocellular carcinoma: a randomized trial. Aliment Pharmacol Ther 2004;19(7):779–88.

96. Poupon RE, Chretien Y, Chazouilleres O, et al. Quality of life in patients with primary biliary cirrhosis. Hepatology 2004;40(2):489–94.

97. Arguedas MR, DeLawrence TG, McGuire BM. Influence of hepatic encephalopathy on health-related quality of life in patients with cirrhosis. Dig Dis Sci 2003;48(8):1622–6.

98. Wunsch E, Szymanik B, Post M, et al. Minimal hepatic encephalopathy does not impair health-related quality of life in patients with cirrhosis: a prospective study. Liver Int 2011;31(7):980–4.

99. Moscucci F, Nardelli S, Pentassuglio I, et al. Previous overt hepatic encephalopathy rather than minimal hepatic encephalopathy impairs health-related quality of life in cirrhotic patients. Liver Int 2011;31(10):1505–10.

100. Bajaj JS, Saeian K, Schubert CM, et al. Minimal hepatic encephalopathy is associated with motor vehicle crashes: the reality beyond the driving test. Hepatology 2009;50(4):1175–83.

101. Bajaj JS. Minimal hepatic encephalopathy matters in daily life. World J Gastroenterol 2008;14(23):3609–15.

102. Montomoli J, Holland-Fischer P, Bianchi G, et al. Body composition changes after transjugular intrahepatic portosystemic shunt in patients with cirrhosis. World J Gastroenterol 2010;16(3):348–53.
103. Campillo B, Bories PN, Pornin B, et al. Influence of liver failure, ascites, and energy expenditure on the response to oral nutrition in alcoholic liver cirrhosis. Nutrition 1997;13(7–8):613–21.
104. Ndraha S, Hasan I, Simadibrata M. The effect of L-ornithine L-aspartate and branch chain amino acids on encephalopathy and nutritional status in liver cirrhosis with malnutrition. Acta Med Indones 2011;43(1):18–22.
105. Dong MH, Saab S. Complications of cirrhosis. Dis Mon 2008;54(7):445–56.
106. Moller S, Bendtsen F, Christensen E, et al. Prognostic variables in patients with cirrhosis and oesophageal varices without prior bleeding. J Hepatol 1994;21(6): 940–6.
107. Olde Damink SW, Jalan R, Dejong CH. Interorgan ammonia trafficking in liver disease. Metab Brain Dis 2009;24(1):169–81.
108. Soros P, Bottcher J, Weissenborn K, et al. Malnutrition and hypermetabolism are not risk factors for the presence of hepatic encephalopathy: a cross-sectional study. J Gastroenterol Hepatol 2008;23(4):606–10.
109. Kalaitzakis E, Bjornsson E. Hepatic encephalopathy in patients with liver cirrhosis: is there a role of malnutrition? World J Gastroenterol 2008;14(21):3438–9.
110. Periyalwar P, Dasarathy J, Tsien C, et al. Sarcopenia of cirrhosis results in more severe and frequent episodes of hepatic encephalopathy. Hepatology 2011. [Epub ahead of print].
111. Dasarathy S, Mullen KD, Conjeevaram HS, et al. Preservation of portal pressure improves growth and metabolic profile in the male portacaval-shunted rat. Dig Dis Sci 2002;47(9):1936–42.
112. Dasarathy S, Yang Y, Muc S, et al. Ammonia causes elevated skeletal muscle myostatin and reduced myoblast proliferation. Hepatology 2009. [Epub ahead of print].
113. McCullough AJ, Mullen KD, Kalhan SC. Defective nonoxidative leucine degradation and endogenous leucine flux in cirrhosis during an amino acid infusion. Hepatology 1998;28(5):1357–64.
114. Kung T, Springer J, Doehner W, et al. Novel treatment approaches to cachexia and sarcopenia: highlights from the 5th Cachexia Conference. Expert Opin Investig Drugs 2010;19(4):579–85.
115. Glass DJ. Skeletal muscle hypertrophy and atrophy signaling pathways. Int J Biochem Cell Biol 2005;37(10):1974–84.
116. Wagers AJ, Conboy IM. Cellular and molecular signatures of muscle regeneration: current concepts and controversies in adult myogenesis. Cell 2005;122(5):659–67.
117. Le GF, Rudnicki MA. Skeletal muscle satellite cells and adult myogenesis. Curr Opin Cell Biol 2007;19(6):628–33.
118. Garlick PJ, McNurlan MA, Essen P, et al. Measurement of tissue protein synthesis rates in vivo: a critical analysis of contrasting methods. Am J Physiol 1994;266(3 Pt 1):E287–97.
119. Welle S, Bhatt K, Pinkert CA. Myofibrillar protein synthesis in myostatin-deficient mice. Am J Physiol Endocrinol Metab 2006;290(3):E409–15.
120. Mullen KD, Denne SC, McCullough AJ, et al. Leucine metabolism in stable cirrhosis. Hepatology 1986;6(4):622–30.
121. Tessari P, Barazzoni R, Kiwanuka E, et al. Impairment of albumin and whole body postprandial protein synthesis in compensated liver cirrhosis. Am J Physiol Endocrinol Metab 2002;282(2):E304–11.

122. Tessari P, Inchiostro S, Barazzoni R, et al. Fasting and postprandial phenylalanine and leucine kinetics in liver cirrhosis. Am J Physiol 1994;267(1 Pt 1):E140–9.

123. Morrison WL, Bouchier IA, Gibson JN, et al. Skeletal muscle and whole-body protein turnover in cirrhosis. Clin Sci (Lond) 1990;78(6):613–9.

124. Tessari P, Biolo G, Inchiostro S, et al. Leucine and phenylalanine kinetics in compensated liver cirrhosis: effects of insulin. Gastroenterology 1993;104(6): 1712–21.

125. Tugtekin I, Wachter U, Barth E, et al. Phenylalanine kinetics in healthy volunteers and liver cirrhotics: implications for the phenylalanine breath test. Am J Physiol Endocrinol Metab 2002;283(6):E1223–31.

126. McCullough AJ, Tavill AS. Disordered energy and protein metabolism in liver disease. Semin Liver Dis 1991;11(4):265–77.

127. Guillet C, Boirie Y, Walrand S. An integrative approach to in-vivo protein synthesis measurement: from whole tissue to specific proteins. Curr Opin Clin Nutr Metab Care 2004;7(5):531–8.

128. Holecek M, Skopec F, Sprongl L. Protein metabolism in cirrhotic rats: effect of dietary restriction. Ann Nutr Metab 1995;39(6):346–54.

129. Lundborg H, Hamberger A. Effects of portacaval anastomosis on liver and brain protein synthesis in rats. Surgery 1977;82(5):643–7.

130. Dunlop DS, Kaufman H, Zanchin G, et al. Protein synthesis rates in rats with portacaval shunts. J Neurochem 1984;43(5):1487–9.

131. Wang YY, Lin SY, Chuang YH, et al. Protein nitration is associated with increased proteolysis in skeletal muscle of bile duct ligation-induced cirrhotic rats. Metabolism 2010;59(4):468–72.

132. Mizushima N, Komatsu M. Autophagy: renovation of cells and tissues. Cell 2011;147(4):728–41.

133. Masiero E, Agatea L, Mammucari C, et al. Autophagy is required to maintain muscle mass. Cell Metab 2009;10(6):507–15.

134. Kandarian SC, Jackman RW. Intracellular signaling during skeletal muscle atrophy. Muscle Nerve 2006;33(2):155–65.

135. Machida S, Booth FW. Regrowth of skeletal muscle atrophied from inactivity. Med Sci Sports Exerc 2004;36(1):52–9.

136. Bornemann A, Maier F, Kuschel R. Satellite cells as players and targets in normal and diseased muscle. Neuropediatrics 1999;30(4):167–75.

137. Hepple RT. Dividing to keep muscle together: the role of satellite cells in aging skeletal muscle. Sci Aging Knowledge Environ 2006;2006(3):e3.

138. Anthony JC, Yoshizawa F, Anthony TG, et al. Leucine stimulates translation initiation in skeletal muscle of postabsorptive rats via a rapamycin-sensitive pathway. J Nutr 2000;130(10):2413–9.

139. Bodine SC, Stitt TN, Gonzalez M, et al. Akt/mTOR pathway is a crucial regulator of skeletal muscle hypertrophy and can prevent muscle atrophy in vivo. Nat Cell Biol 2001;3(11):1014–9.

140. Lokireddy S, Mouly V, Butler-Browne G, et al. Myostatin promotes the wasting of human myoblast cultures through promoting ubiquitin-proteasome pathway-mediated loss of sarcomeric proteins. Am J Physiol Cell Physiol 2011;301(6): C1316–24.

141. Zimmers TA, Davies MV, Koniaris LG, et al. Induction of cachexia in mice by systemically administered myostatin. Science 2002;296(5572):1486–8.

142. Morissette MR, Cook SA, Buranasombati C, et al. Myostatin inhibits IGF-I-induced myotube hypertrophy through Akt. Am J Physiol Cell Physiol 2009; 297(5):C1124–32.

143. Trendelenburg AU, Meyer A, Rohner D, et al. Myostatin reduces Akt/TORC1/ p70S6K signaling, inhibiting myoblast differentiation and myotube size. Am J Physiol Cell Physiol 2009;296(6):C1258–70.

144. Lee JY, Hopkinson NS, Kemp PR. Myostatin induces autophagy in skeletal muscle in vitro. Biochem Biophys Res Commun 2011;415(4):632–6.

145. Goldspink G. Age-related muscle loss and progressive dysfunction in mechano-sensitive growth factor signaling. Ann N Y Acad Sci 2004;1019:294–8.

146. Bush JA, Kimball SR, O'Connor PM, et al. Translational control of protein synthesis in muscle and liver of growth hormone-treated pigs. Endocrinology 2003;144(4):1273–83.

147. Latres E, Amini AR, Amini AA, et al. Insulin-like growth factor-1 (IGF-1) inversely regulates atrophy-induced genes via the phosphatidylinositol 3-kinase/Akt/ mammalian target of rapamycin (PI3K/Akt/mTOR) pathway. J Biol Chem 2005; 280(4):2737–44.

148. Berger MJ, Doherty TJ. Sarcopenia: prevalence, mechanisms, and functional consequences. Interdiscip Top Gerontol 2010;37:94–114.

149. Doherty TJ. Invited review: aging and sarcopenia. J Appl Physiol 2003;95(4): 1717–27.

150. Pagadala M, Dasarathy S, Eghtesad B, et al. Posttransplant metabolic syndrome: an epidemic waiting to happen. Liver Transpl 2009;15(12):1662–70.

151. Guillet C, Boirie Y. Insulin resistance: a contributing factor to age-related muscle mass loss? Diabetes Metab 2005;31(Spec No 2):5S20–6.

152. Michel RN, Chin ER, Chakkalakal JV, et al. Ca2+/calmodulin-based signalling in the regulation of the muscle fibre phenotype and its therapeutic potential via modulation of utrophin A and myostatin expression. Appl Physiol Nutr Metab 2007;32(5):921–9.

153. Sakuma K, Nakao R, Aoi W, et al. Cyclosporin A treatment upregulates Id1 and Smad3 expression and delays skeletal muscle regeneration. Acta Neuropathol 2005;110(3):269–80.

154. Lipina C, Kendall H, McPherron AC, et al. Mechanisms involved in the enhancement of mammalian target of rapamycin signalling and hypertrophy in skeletal muscle of myostatin-deficient mice. FEBS Lett 2010;584(11):2403–8.

155. Scolapio JS, Bowen J, Stoner G, et al. Substrate oxidation in patients with cirrhosis: comparison with other nutritional markers. JPEN J Parenter Enteral Nutr 2000;24(3):150–3.

156. Cabre E, Gonzalez-Huix F, bad-Lacruz A, et al. Effect of total enteral nutrition on the short-term outcome of severely malnourished cirrhotics. A randomized controlled trial. Gastroenterology 1990;98(3):715–20.

157. Plauth M, Cabre E, Riggio O, et al. ESPEN guidelines on enteral nutrition: liver disease. Clin Nutr 2006;25(2):285–94.

158. Bucuvalas JC, Cutfield W, Horn J, et al. Resistance to the growth-promoting and metabolic effects of growth hormone in children with chronic liver disease. J Pediatr 1990;117(3):397–402.

159. Moller S, Becker U, Gronbaek M, et al. Short-term effect of recombinant human growth hormone in patients with alcoholic cirrhosis. J Hepatol 1994;21(5):710–7.

160. Donaghy A, Ross R, Wicks C, et al. Growth hormone therapy in patients with cirrhosis: a pilot study of efficacy and safety. Gastroenterology 1997;113(5): 1617–22.

161. Wallace JD, bbott-Johnson WJ, Crawford DH, et al. GH treatment in adults with chronic liver disease: a randomized, double-blind, placebo-controlled, cross-over study. J Clin Endocrinol Metab 2002;87(6):2751–9.

162. Cabral CM, Burns DL. Low-protein diets for hepatic encephalopathy debunked: let them eat steak. Nutr Clin Pract 2011;26(2):155–9.
163. Gundling F, Seidl H, Pehl C, et al. How close do gastroenterologists follow specific guidelines for nutrition recommendations in liver cirrhosis? A survey of current practice. Eur J Gastroenterol Hepatol 2009;21(7):756–61.
164. Heyman JK, Whitfield CJ, Brock KE, et al. Dietary protein intakes in patients with hepatic encephalopathy and cirrhosis: current practice in NSW and ACT. Med J Aust 2006;185(10):542–3.
165. Kondrup J, Nielsen K, Juul A. Effect of long-term refeeding on protein metabolism in patients with cirrhosis of the liver. Br J Nutr 1997;77(2):197–212.
166. Porter C, Cohen NH. Indirect calorimetry in critically ill patients: role of the clinical dietitian in interpreting results. J Am Diet Assoc 1996;96(1):49–57.
167. Kondrup J, Muller MJ. Energy and protein requirements of patients with chronic liver disease. J Hepatol 1997;27(1):239–47.
168. Nielsen K, Kondrup J, Martinsen L, et al. Long-term oral refeeding of patients with cirrhosis of the liver. Br J Nutr 1995;74(4):557–67.
169. Plauth M, Roske AE, Romaniuk P, et al. Post-feeding hyperammonaemia in patients with transjugular intrahepatic portosystemic shunt and liver cirrhosis: role of small intestinal ammonia release and route of nutrient administration. Gut 2000;46(6):849–55.
170. Swart GR, van den Berg JW, van Vuure JK, et al. Minimum protein requirements in liver cirrhosis determined by nitrogen balance measurements at three levels of protein intake. Clin Nutr 1989;8(6):329–36.
171. Vaisman N, Katzman H, Carmiel-Haggai M, et al. Breakfast improves cognitive function in cirrhotic patients with cognitive impairment. Am J Clin Nutr 2010; 92(1):137–40.
172. Khanna S, Gopalan S. Role of branched-chain amino acids in liver disease: the evidence for and against. Curr Opin Clin Nutr Metab Care 2007;10(3):297–303.
173. Kachaamy T, Bajaj JS. Diet and cognition in chronic liver disease. Curr Opin Gastroenterol 2011;27(2):174–9.
174. Anthony JC, Anthony TG, Kimball SR, et al. Signaling pathways involved in translational control of protein synthesis in skeletal muscle by leucine. J Nutr 2001;131(3):856S–60S.
175. Dreyer HC, Drummond MJ, Pennings B, et al. Leucine-enriched essential amino acid and carbohydrate ingestion following resistance exercise enhances mTOR signaling and protein synthesis in human muscle. Am J Physiol Endocrinol Metab 2008;294(2):E392–400.
176. Drummond MJ, Rasmussen BB. Leucine-enriched nutrients and the regulation of mammalian target of rapamycin signalling and human skeletal muscle protein synthesis. Curr Opin Clin Nutr Metab Care 2008;11(3):222–6.
177. Koopman R, Wagenmakers AJ, Manders RJ, et al. Combined ingestion of protein and free leucine with carbohydrate increases postexercise muscle protein synthesis in vivo in male subjects. Am J Physiol Endocrinol Metab 2005;288(4):E645–53.
178. Katsanos CS, Kobayashi H, Sheffield-Moore M, et al. A high proportion of leucine is required for optimal stimulation of the rate of muscle protein synthesis by essential amino acids in the elderly. Am J Physiol Endocrinol Metab 2006; 291(2):E381–7.
179. Lee SJ, Glass DJ. Treating cancer cachexia to treat cancer. Skelet Muscle 2011; 1(1):2.

180. Rode A, Fourlanos S, Nicoll A. Oral vitamin D replacement is effective in chronic liver disease. Gastroenterol Clin Biol 2010;34(11):618–20.
181. Stamoulis I, Kouraklis G, Theocharis S. Zinc and the liver: an active interaction. Dig Dis Sci 2007;52(7):1595–612.
182. Yoshida Y, Higashi T, Nouso K, et al. Effects of zinc deficiency/zinc supplementation on ammonia metabolism in patients with decompensated liver cirrhosis. Acta Med Okayama 2001;55(6):349–55.
183. Bavdekar A, Bhave S, Pandit A. Nutrition management in chronic liver disease. Indian J Pediatr 2002;69(5):427–31.
184. Crawford BA, Labio ED, Strasser SI, et al. Vitamin D replacement for cirrhosis-related bone disease. Nat Clin Pract Gastroenterol Hepatol 2006;3(12):689–99.
185. Drummond MJ, Dreyer HC, Pennings B, et al. Skeletal muscle protein anabolic response to resistance exercise and essential amino acids is delayed with aging. J Appl Physiol 2008;104(5):1452–61.
186. Wilborn CD, Taylor LW, Greenwood M, et al. Effects of different intensities of resistance exercise on regulators of myogenesis. J Strength Cond Res 2009; 23(8):2179–87.
187. Koopman R, Saris WH, Wagenmakers AJ, et al. Nutritional interventions to promote post-exercise muscle protein synthesis. Sports Med 2007;37(10): 895–906.
188. Garcia-Pagan JC, Santos C, Barbera JA, et al. Physical exercise increases portal pressure in patients with cirrhosis and portal hypertension. Gastroenterology 1996;111(5):1300–6.
189. Garcia PS, Cabbabe A, Kambadur R, et al. Brief-reports: elevated myostatin levels in patients with liver disease: a potential contributor to skeletal muscle wasting. Anesth Analg 2010;111(3):707–9.
190. Harrison J, McKiernan J, Neuberger JM. A prospective study on the effect of recipient nutritional status on outcome in liver transplantation. Transpl Int 1997;10(5):369–74.
191. Stephenson GR, Moretti EW, El-Moalem H, et al. Malnutrition in liver transplant patients: preoperative subjective global assessment is predictive of outcome after liver transplantation. Transplantation 2001;72(4):666–70.
192. Campillo B, Richardet JP, Scherman E, et al. Evaluation of nutritional practice in hospitalized cirrhotic patients: results of a prospective study. Nutrition 2003; 19(6):515–21.

Hepatic Encephalopathy After Transjugular Intrahepatic Portosystemic Shunt

Oliviero Riggio, MD*, Silvia Nardelli, MD, Federica Moscucci, MD,
Chiara Pasquale, MD, Lorenzo Ridola, MD, Manuela Merli, MD

KEYWORDS

- Hepatic encephalopathy • Portal hypertension
- Transjugular intrahepatic portosystemic shunt

Transjugular intrahepatic portosystemic shunt (TIPS) has been used since more than 20 years to treat some of the complications of portal hypertension, especially variceal bleeding and ascites refractory to conventional therapy. Since the first description, the indications for the procedure have progressively expanded and, today, the role of TIPS in the treatment of portal hypertension continues to evolve. In 2009, the American Association for the Study of Liver Disease Practice Guidelines for the use of TIPS in the management of portal hypertension have been updated,[1] and further recommendations can be found in the Baveno V Consensus Conference.[2] The technical details of the procedure have been extensively described.[3–6] TIPS establishes a communication between the portal and hepatic veins, inducing the blood to shift from the splanchnic circulation into the systemic vascular bed with the aim of decompressing the portal venous system, and avoids the major complications of portal hypertension (**Fig. 1**). At the same time, the shunt of the portal blood into the systemic circulation is the cause of one of the major complications of the procedure: the so-called post-TIPS hepatic encephalopathy (HE).

HE is a neurologic syndrome characterized by alterations in the patient's mental state (impaired consciousness and/or inappropriate behavior) of different degree (from minor alterations to coma) and abnormalities in neuromuscular function.[7] HE may be a consequence of pure liver failure, as in patients with fulminant hepatitis, or of the combination of liver failure and portal-systemic shunting, as in patients with liver

Department of Clinical Medicine, Centre for the Diagnosis and Treatment of Portal Hypertension, Sapienza University of Rome, Viale dell'Università 37, 00185 Rome, Italy
* Corresponding author.
E-mail address: oliviero.riggio@uniroma1.it

Clin Liver Dis 16 (2012) 133–146
doi:10.1016/j.cld.2011.12.008
1089-3261/12/$ – see front matter © 2012 Elsevier Inc. All rights reserved.

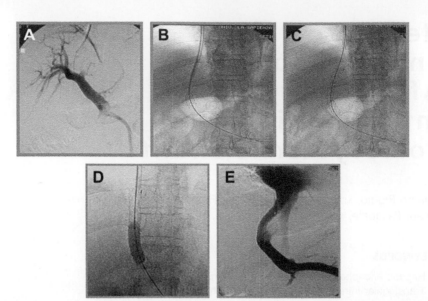

Fig. 1. Different phases of a TIPS implantation with polytetrafluoroethylene-covered stents. (*A*) Portal vein puncture. (*B*) Release of the uncovered portion within the portal vein by withdrawing the introducer. (*C*) Release of the covered portion within the hepatic tract. (*D*) Balloon dilatation of the stent after the release. (*E*) Angiographic appearance.

cirrhosis. Several clinical and pathophysiologic observations suggest the importance of portal-systemic shunts in the development of HE. In patients with noncirrhotic portal hypertension with minimal alterations of liver function, the presence of large portal-systemic shunts may be associated with neurologic abnormalities,[8,9] abnormal ammonia levels, and magnetic resonance spectroscopy pattern[10] similar to that observed in cirrhotic patients with HE.[11] In liver cirrhosis, the relationship between portal-systemic shunting and HE is less clear because the shunts occur in patients with a concomitant significant reduction of liver function and perfusion. However, in cirrhotic patients, HE may develop immediately after a surgical[12,13] or radiologic portacaval shunt,[14–16] and a relationship between the size of the anastomosis and the incidence of HE may be demonstrated.[13–17] Post-TIPS HE, resistant to medical treatment, may ameliorate by reducing the shunt diameter.[18]

When TIPS was initially proposed, it was claimed that the optimal calibration of the shunt could allow an adequate reduction of portal hypertension, avoiding, at the same time, the occurrence of HE. However, several clinical observations have shown that HE occurred rather frequently after TIPS,[14–16,19] and HE has become an important issue to be taken into consideration in TIPS candidates and a problem to be faced after the procedure. To date, with the use of the new polytetrafluoroethylene (PTFE)-covered stents that have reduced significantly the incidence of shunt insufficiency,[20] the main problem in the long-term management of patients submitted to TIPS is probably HE.

Two main phenomena are likely to be related to post-TIPS HE: portal blood diversion from the liver due to portacaval shunting and the decrease in liver metabolic capacity. The entity of portal diversion is variable and dependent on the stent diameter and the portosystemic gradient after the procedure.[21] The liver metabolic capacity depends on the degree of liver failure before TIPS, which, however, may be further reduced by the procedure.

INCIDENCE OF POST-TIPS HE

The current knowledge about the incidence of post-TIPS HE derives from the prospective studies available. Some discrepancies, however, may arise due to the method used for classifying and staging the syndrome. In fact, some studies considered the overall episodes of HE, whereas others have only considered the new or worsened HE episodes. Some investigators have selected the episodes that occurred "without an evident precipitating cause"[22,23] and others only those leading the patients to hospitalization.

The overall incidence of post-TIPS HE ranges between 25% and 45%, however, when only the new or worsened HE is considered, depending on how many patients with previous HE were observed, a lower percentage of HE was found (13–36%).[14–16,24,25]

The incidence of post-TIPS HE can also be derived by the randomized controlled trials (RCTs) in which TIPS was compared with standard nonderivative therapy for the prevention of variceal rebleeding[22,26–31] or the treatment of refractory ascites.[32–37] In the RCTs for the prevention of variceal rebleeding, the incidence of post-TIPS HE was significantly higher than that reported in patients submitted to nonderivative treatment. This observation was not confirmed in the trials comparing TIPS with large-volume paracentesis for intractable ascites in which the rate of HE was similar in the 2 groups of patients, probably because of the very high incidence of HE, independent of TIPS, in patients with very advanced liver disease and refractory ascites. However, even in this kind of patients, severe HE was more frequent in those submitted to TIPS than in those treated with repeated paracentesis. Chronic/recurrent HE was reported in the TIPS group only (**Table 1**).

CHARACTERISTICS OF POST-TIPS HE

When bare metal stents were used for TIPS insertion, HE tends to be particularly frequent during the first months after TIPS and less common with time. This behavior is thought to be due to the development of shunt stenosis, which, even when not clinically overt (in this case the shunt is usually revised), can progressively reduce the amount of the portal blood shunted.[14–16,19] With the new PTFE-covered endoprostheses, the number of shunt stenoses is considerably reduced.[20] Thus, a possible increase in the risk of HE related to the use of covered stents has been suggested.[38]

The studies on the incidence and the characteristic of HE after TIPS with covered stents are few. In studies in which a direct comparison between covered and bare stents was made, the incidence[20] of post-TIPS HE was actually reduced[20] or at least not increased[39,40] in patients treated with the new endoprostheses. One possible explanation for this observation is that the reduced number of shunt revision (dilatation or restenting) that is performed in patients treated with the covered stent may reduce the episodes of HE that may occur immediately after a shunt revision.

Another concern about HE in patients treated with PTFE-covered stents was the possibility of an increased number of patients with recurrent or persistent HE or the possibility that the occurrence of HE was not only confined to the first postoperative period. To test this hypothesis, we analyzed the variations of HE frequency along time by using a multiple events per subjects Cox model in 78 consecutive cirrhotic patients referred to our unit in whom TIPS was performed with PTFE-covered stent grafts (**Fig. 2**).[41] This analysis (in which not only the first episode of HE but also the others occurring during the follow-up have been considered) suggests that the estimated cumulative number of HE events in patients with an initial HE episode remains constant over time. This behavior seems to be different from what has been described in patients submitted to TIPS with traditional bare stents. In addition, with the covered stent, recurrent/persistent HE refractory to standard treatments may also occur with

Table 1
Incidence rate of post-TIPS HE in RCTs

RCTs Comparing TIPS vs Nonderivative Treatment	Number of RCTs[a]	Number[a] of Patients		Number[a] of Patients (%) with HE		Number[a] of Patients (%) with Chronic/Recurrent HE	
		TIPS	Controls	TIPS	Controls	TIPS	Controls
On variceal rebleeding[b]	14	516	515	172 (33)	97 (19)	10 (1.9)	4 (0.7)
1. Cabrera et al,[22] 1996	—	31	32	10	4	3	0
2. Rossle et al,[26] 1997	—	61	65	22	12	2	2
3. Jalan et al,[27] 1997	—	31	27	11[c]	3[c]	1[d]	0
4. Sanyal et al,[28] 1997	—	41	39	12	5	—	—
5. Cello et al,[29] 1997	—	24	25	12	11	—	—
6. Sauer et al,[30] 1997	—	42	41	12	5	—	—
7. Merli et al,[31] 1998	—	38	43	21	10	—	—
8. Garcia Pagan et al,[59] 2010	—	32	31	8	12	1	1
9. Lo et al,[60] 2007	—	35	37	10	1	—	—
10. Sauer et al,[61] 2002	—	43	42	17	9	—	—
11. Gülberg et al,[62] 2002	—	28	26	2	1	—	—
12. Escorsell et al,[63] 2002	—	47	44	15	2	—	—
13. Pomier-Layrargues et al,[64] 2001	—	41	39	15	16	—	—
14. Garcia Villareal et al,[65] 1999	—	22	24	5	6	3	1
On refractory ascites[a]	6	192	198	102 (53)	63 (32)	7 (3.6)	3 (1.5)
1. Rössle et al,[33] 2000	—	29	31	15	11	1[d]	2[d]
2. Sanyal et al,[35] 2003	—	52	57	20	12	—	—
3. Ginès et al,[34] 2002	—	35	35	27	23	—	—
4. Salerno et al,[36] 2004	—	33	33	20	13	1[d]	0
5. Lebrec et al,[32] 1996	—	13	12	3	0	2	0
6. Narahara et al,[37] 2011	—	30	30	17	4	3	1

[a] In patients submitted for TIPS for the treatment of refractory ascites, the difference in the incidence rate of HE of any degree was similar (not significant) in 4 RCTs.[33–36] However, the incidence rate of severe HE was significantly higher in the TIPS group in 3[34–36] of 5 RCTs (Rössle et al,[33] 2000, no data on severity of HE).
[b] In patients submitted for TIPS for the prevention of variceal rebleeding, the difference in the incidence rate of HE was significantly higher in the TIPS group in 7[22,26,27,30,31,61,63] of 13 RCTs.
[c] Only patients free from HE at TIPS insertion.
[d] Needed shunt reduction.

a rate (8%–10%) similar to that observed in patients treated with bare stents. Therefore, although the incidence of HE seemed to be not increased by the use of covered stent, post-TIPS HE is actually still regrettably frequent with the new covered stents as it was with traditional bare stents.

PREDICTORS OF POST-TIPS HE

Previous HE was found to be a very strong predictor of post-TIPS; almost all patients who previously had recurrent HE presented with encephalopathy after TIPS, and, thus,

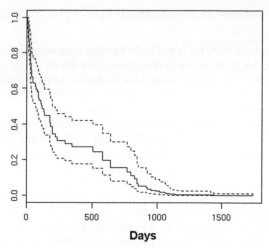

Fig. 2. Survival curve of HE repeated episodes in the whole population of 78 patients treated with TIPS constructed with PTFE-covered stents. At least 1 episode of HE occurred in 35 of the 78 patients. The total number of HE episodes in the 35 of 78 patients during the whole follow-up period was 89. Fifty-five percent of the episodes were graded as severe. (*Data from* Riggio O, Angeloni S, Salvatori FM, et al. Incidence, natural history, and risk factors of hepatic encephalopathy after transjugular intrahepatic portosystemic shunt with polytetrafluoroethylene-covered stent grafts. Am J Gastroenterol 2008;103:2738–46.)

this kind of HE should be probably considered as a contraindication to TIPS.[42] However, it should be noted that patients with a single episode of HE due to variceal bleeding may not be at risk of HE after TIPS. Others predictors of post-TIPS HE identified were age,[16,26] low portacaval pressure gradient (PPG),[16,43] and high Child-Pugh score. These factors were identified as the most robust HE predictors in a systematic review recently conducted.[44] Further factors associated with post-TIPS HE were high creatinine levels, low serum sodium concentration,[41,45] and minimal HE before TIPS.[46]

In patients treated with PTFE-covered stents,[41] older age, high creatinine levels, and low serum sodium and albumin levels were the parameters related to the development of post-TIPS HE. It should be noted that in this study patients with previous HE were excluded. A high creatinine level was the only parameter independently related to the development of chronic/recurrent post-TIPS refractory HE.

Taking into account the earlier observations, the risk of post-TIPS HE can be segregated as follows:

1. Patients at high risk of post-TIPS HE are those who suffered from more than 1 episode of HE in the past. In these patients, TIPS procedure should be considered as contraindicated and used with caution only when all other measures to treat complications of portal hypertension have failed and probably only if the patients have variceal bleeding and there are no therapeutic alternatives. In these patients, multiple episodes of HE are expected after TIPS.
2. Patients at medium risk are those older than 60 years (or than 65 years in other studies) and with other risk factors such as severe liver insufficiency. These patients should be treated with TIPS according to the general indications taking into account that HE will probably represent a problem.
3. Patients at low risk have preserved liver function, are younger than 65 years, and have never experienced previous episodes of HE. Although an episode of post-TIPS HE

may present in these patients, the episodes (or episode) will probably not be severe or long lasting.

Chronic/recurrent refractory HE is the most serious concern regarding patients who are to be submitted to TIPS. In the largest described series of patients (38 patients) with this complication,[47] the only apparent risk factor for refractory HE was the greater age of patients with refractory HE compared with those without. Other factors, such as the presence or absence of pre-TIPS HE or the final portal pressure gradient after TIPS, were not different compared with other patients undergoing TIPS and not developing refractory HE. In patients without HE before TIPS treated with PTFE-covered stent the only factor associated with the development of refractory HE was a creatinine level greater than normal values before TIPS insertion (odds ratio, 4.63; 95% confidence limit, 1.1–19.3; $P = .04$).[41] The optimal cutoff was determined as 1.1 mg/dL, with patients above that threshold having a probability 12.05 times higher of developing refractory HE. However, if this criterion is used for classifying a patient as high risk for developing refractory HE, it is expected that 83.3% of true developers will be correctly identified, but 25% of patients who would have not developed the refractory HE will be wrongly classified as at high risk. In other words, 1 of 4 patients might not be submitted to TIPS because of the erroneous prediction of refractory HE after TIPS.[41] Therefore, the risk factors for this important complication still need to be better clarified.

PREVENTION OF POST-TIPS HE

Because patients submitted to TIPS are at high risk of developing post-TIPS HE, and because selecting only patients at low risk of developing this complication to undergo the procedure is not always possible, a pharmacologic treatment to prevent the occurrence of HE would be very much appreciated. However, to date, there is no evidence of efficacious prophylactic treatments of HE after a TIPS. The only randomized controlled trial performed for this aim failed to show any beneficial effect of drugs commonly used in the treatment of HE. In fact in that study, the incidence of HE within 1 month after TIPS construction was not significantly reduced by the administration of either nonabsorbable disaccharides or low-absorbable antibiotics (rifaximin) compared with that observed in the no-treatment arm.[46] Recently, these 2 treatments were shown to prevent the occurrence of HE in patients not submitted to TIPS but at high risk for HE, such as cirrhotic patients with a recent episode of HE. It is not easy to explain why the same treatment is able to prevent HE in cirrhotic patients and not in patients submitted to TIPS. Although the hypothesis involving the primary role of gut-derived neurotoxins, especially ammonia, in the pathogenesis of HE in patients with or without TIPS is shareable, we believe that opening a TIPS constitutes a completely different scenario that makes HE particularly difficult to be prevented. In fact, after TIPS, further compromise of first-pass hepatic clearance of ammonia is to be expected. In addition, the increases in splanchnic blood flow occurring after TIPS may enhance the delivery of ammonia into the systemic circulation. Another factor to be considered is the upregulation of intestinal glutaminase activity, which has been reported after experimental portosystemic shunt procedures.[48] This enzyme is responsible for the large amount of ammonia generated by the small intestine. Accordingly, one might anticipate that in the immediate aftermath of a TIPS procedure, more intense HE therapy might be needed to prevent overt episodes of HE than in patients not submitted to TIPS.

Another possible approach would be to avoid the excessive diversion of portal blood by using stents with smaller diameters, at least in patients at high risk of post-TIPS HE.

Recently an RCT was performed to assess the efficacy of PTFE stents with different diameters (10 vs 8 mm) on the incidence of post-TIPS HE. However, the trial was stopped because the stents with smaller diameter were unable to control the complications of portal hypertension.[49] Another interesting hypothesis is to use adjustable stent systems to modulate the PPG to reduce the incidence of HE. An adjustable stent device developed specifically for TIPS construction is not available, but the stent diameter can be modulated by implanting a balloon-expandable stent graft inside the original stent used for TIPS implantation. A difficulty is that the value of PPG required to avoid the occurrence of HE is unknown. Moreover, immediately after the procedure, the amount of blood reaching the heart increases rapidly, with a consequent increase in the right atrium and central venous pressure.[50,51] The myocardial adaptation to this new hemodynamic condition may occur in a variable time.[50,51] Consequently, the PPG value measured immediately after TIPS opening does not remain stable over time. It is therefore difficult to be able to modulate an instable PPG to reach an unknown value. For these reasons, we believe that HE will remain a major problem after TIPS until new treatments for HE prevention will become available.

TREATMENT OF POST-TIPS HE
Episodic HE

Episodes of HE after TIPS can be treated traditionally. The cornerstones of the treatment of this type of HE are the identification and treatment of the precipitating event and the general support of the patients. This includes the prevention of falls or body injuries in disorientated patients, care of bladder and bowel functions, care of intravenous lines, monitoring of fluid balance, monitoring of blood glycemia and electrolyte levels such as of arterial blood gases, correction of acid/base disorders, blood pressure monitoring, and avoidance of aspiration pneumonia. The nutritional status of the patient should also be taken into consideration. Some strategies commonly applied to stop the precipitating event are to treat infections by appropriate antibiotic therapies, constipation by cathartic and/or bowel enema, and electrolyte abnormalities by discontinuing diuretics and correcting hypokalemia or hyperkalemia. Stopping the diuretics, treating the dehydration, and discontinuing the nephrotoxic drugs should correct deterioration of the renal function, if present.[52]

Chronic Recurrent HE

Chronic recurrent HE refractory to standard treatment is, in our opinion, the most important problem faced when a patients has to be treated with TIPS. In some cases, the occurrence of this complication may deeply reduce the patient's quality of life and the cure may be worse than the disease. In patients with refractory ascites, for example, the repeated paracentesis may not limit the patient's autonomy as TIPS-induced refractory HE.

Chronic recurrent HE refractory to standard treatment can be treated by reducing the diameter of the stent or by occluding the shunt. In fact, HE ameliorated in most patients submitted to this shunt revision. However, the procedure is not without dangers and may not solve the problem in all patients, and the complications of portal hypertension, such as varices or refractory ascites, which were supposed to be managed by the TIPS, may recur as a consequence of shunt reduction or occlusion. Therefore, the decision of revising the shunt should be taken with caution, on a strict definition of refractory HE and only in patients free of portal hypertension before the revision (**Table 2**). Moreover, ideally, the shunt should be revised only in patients in whom the causal relationship between the shunt and HE is likely, avoiding to perform

Table 2
Factors influencing the decision of reducing the diameter of the shunt in patients with chronic/recurrent refractory post-TIPS HE

Factors	Suggestions
Strict definition of refractory HE	• At least 3 episodes of nonprecipitant-induced severe encephalopathy requiring hospitalization in the last 3 mo despite continuous treatment with nonabsorbable disaccharides or • Persistent HE, defined as the presence of a continuously detectable altered mental state despite protein restriction to 1 g/kg of body weight and treatment with nonabsorbable disaccharides
Causal relationship between the shunt and HE	Likely if • Short distance between the onset of refractory HE and TIPS implantation • Low portal-systemic gradient supporting the importance of blood diversionUnlikely if • Clinical signs of portal hypertension before revision • Deterioration of liver function after TIPS
Low risk of variceal bleeding	• Check the varices before and after the shunt revision • Start preventive treatment after the revision

the procedure in those with chronic refractory HE due to liver failure. Even this one is not an easy decision. Although the procedure adopted for the reduction of the diameter permits the portal pressure modulation, it is very difficult to establish which portosystemic pressure gradient values should be reached to avoid further episodes of HE as well as events eventually occurring after the recurrence of portal hypertension.

The most relevant studies[41,47,53–57] reporting the data and the outcome of patients with chronic/recurrent post-TIPS HE submitted to shunt reduction or occlusion are summarized in **Table 3**. Several techniques to modulate the shunt diameter have been described. The details on how the shunt can be reduced or occluded are not the object of this article.

A strict definition of post-TIPS refractory HE is not available. Refractory HE was defined as clinically significant if it interfered with the day-to-day activities of patients and/or led to repeated hospital admissions.[47] We performed the shunt revision after at least 3 episodes of nonprecipitant-induced severe encephalopathy requiring hospitalization in the last 3 months despite continuous treatment with nonabsorbable disaccharides or when there was a persistent HE, defined as the presence of a continuously detectable altered mental state with further episodic deterioration despite protein restriction to 1 g/kg of body weight and treatment with nonabsorbable disaccharides.[41] Several complications have been related to the procedure. Compared with shunt reduction, occlusion of the shunt involves a higher risk of complications (including intestinal infarction due to thrombosis of the superior mesenteric vein) and deaths[47] and, therefore, should be avoided. The recurrence of symptomatic portal hypertension (varices and ascites) was also described in all series, and deaths related to variceal bleeding occurred. In our opinion, the risk of bleeding from varices should be carefully assessed in all patients undergoing shunt reduction before and after the procedure, and endoscopy should always be repeated early and then periodically after shunt revision to start timely the prevention of variceal bleeding. In some cases, ascites recurred after the shunt reduction and again became refractory to medical therapy.

Table 3
Main studies reporting the effect of shunt reduction in patients with chronic/recurrent refractory post-TIPS HE

Studies	Number of Patients with Refractory HE/Treated with TIPS	Child-Pugh Class (A/B/C)	Number of Patients in Whom Condition Improved	Adverse Events After TIPS Reduction	Pre-PPG (mm Hg)	Post-PPG (mm Hg)
Cookson et al,[53] 2011	8/not reported	B: 3 C: 5	5	Bleeding: 3 Deaths: 2	4.9 ± 3.6	10.5 ± 3.9
Fanelli et al,[54] 2009	12/189	A: 1 B: 5 C: 6	12	Ascites: 1 OLT: 1 Deaths: 4	6.6 ± 2.69	15.1 ± 3.4
Riggio et al,[41] 2008	6/78	—	6	Ascites: 1 Death for bleeding: 1	5.5 ± 2.1	14.7 ± 1.9
Chung et al,[55] 2008	4/113	C: 4	4	—	—	
Maleux et al,[56] 2007	16/266	A: 2 B: 13 C: 1	10	Ascites: 1 Bleeding: 1 OLT: 1	5.25 ± 2.4	11 ± 3.1
Maleux et al,[56] 2007	17/317	A: 3 B: 7 C: 7	13	Ascites: 1 Hydrothorax: 1	6.3 ± 2.4	11.9 ± 3.2
Kochar et al,[47] 2006	38/733	—	21	Bleeding: 3 Ascites: 3 Deaths: 3	—	—
Kerlan et al,[57] 1995	5/not reported	—	4	Bleeding: 1	—	—

Abbreviation: OLT, orthotopic liver transplantation.

Post-TIPS refractory HE does not ameliorate in all patients submitted to shunt reduction/occlusion. In nonresponding patients, probably the deterioration of the liver function is more important than the portal blood diversion; it is to be confirmed that the refractory HE is causally related to the excessive blood diversion and not to liver deterioration. In theory, refractory HE occurring immediately after a TIPS can be probably attributed to the excessive shunt diversion more that that occurring several months after TIPS implantation. However, in some patients, refractory HE developed for the first time after 20 months after TIPS. Although in these cases liver deterioration might have contributed to the onset of HE, the reduction of shunt diameter led to its resolution in these patients also. A very low portal-systemic gradient may support the importance of blood diversion and may make the resolution of HE after that shunt reduction more likely. Once the decision of revising the shunt is taken, the evaluation of the portal-systemic gradient should be done and the procedure should be avoided in patients with a gradient suggesting that blood diversion is not excessive. However, the predictive value of a short distance between the onset of refractory HE and TIPS implantation and of the low portal-systemic gradient before the shunt reduction on the amelioration of refractory post-TIPS HE is not faultless.

SUMMARY

Post-TIPS HE still remains a major unresolved issue because no efficacious strategy has been able to reduce the incidence of this condition that to date so negatively affects patients' quality of life. Thus, a careful and evidence-based indication to TIPS insertion remains mandatory. According to us, once the decision to perform a TIPS has been carefully taken, the patient should be informed that episodic HE is likely to occur at least once after the procedure and that, although infrequently, refractory HE may also occur. Although this latter severe complication of TIPS can be managed by reducing the stent diameter, this operation is not free of risks. In patients with refractory ascites in which TIPS and repeated paracentesis are equivalent in terms of survival,[58] patient's informed preference should be taken into consideration.

REFERENCES

1. Boyer TD, Haskal ZJ. AASLD practice guidelines: the role of transjugular intrahepatic portosystemic shunt (TIPS) in the management of portal hypertension. Hepatology 2010;51:1–16.
2. de Franchis R, Baveno V Faculty. Revising consensus in portal hypertension: report of the Baveno V consensus workshop on methodology of diagnosis and therapy in portal hypertension. J Hepatol 2010;53:762–8.
3. DeGasperi A, Corti A, Corso R, et al. Transjugular intrahepatic portosystemic shunt (TIPS): the anesthesiological point of view after 150 procedures managed under total intravenous anesthesia. J Clin Monit Comput 2009;23:341–6.
4. Shiffman ML, Jeffers L, Hoofnagle JH, et al. Role of transjugular intrahepatic portosystemic shunt treatment of portal hypertension and its complication: conference sponsored by the National Digestive Diseases Advisory Board. Hepatology 1995; 22:1591–7.
5. Rösch J, Keller FS. Transjugular intrahepatic portosystemic shunt: present status, comparison with endoscopic therapy and shunt surgery, and future prospectives. World J Surg 2001;25:337–46.
6. Rössle M, Richter GM, Noldge G, et al. New non-operative treatment for variceal haemorrhage. Lancet 1989;2:153.

7. Ferenci P, Lockwood A, Mullen K, et al. Hepatic encephalopathy: definition, nomenclature, diagnosis, and quantification: final report of the working party at the 11th World Congresses of Gastroenterology, Vienna, 1998. Hepatology 2002; 35:716–21.

8. Watanabe A. Portal-systemic encephalopathy in non-cirrhotic patients: classification of clinical types, diagnosis and treatment. J Gastroenterol Hepatol 2000;15: 969–79.

9. Crespin J, Nemcek A, Rehkemper G, et al. Intrahepatic portal-hepatic venous anastomosis: a portal-systemic shunt with neurological repercussions. Am J Gastroenterol 2000;95:1568–71.

10. Minguez B, Garcia Pagan JC, Bosch J, et al. Noncirrhotic portal vein thrombosis exhibits neuropsychological and MR changes consistent with minimal hepatic encephalopathy. Hepatology 2006;43:707–14.

11. Balata S, Olde Damink S, Ferguson K, et al. Induced hyperammonemia alters neuropsychology, brain MR spectroscopy and magnetization transfer in cirrhosis. Hepatology 2003;37:931–9.

12. Klempnaue J, Schrem H. Review: surgical shunts and encephalopathy. Metab Brain Dis 2001;16:21–8.

13. Hanna SS, Smith RB, Henderson JM, et al. Reversal of hepatic encephalopathy after occlusion of total portosystemic shunts. Am J Surg 1981;142:285–9.

14. Sanjal AJ, Freedman A, Shiffman ML, et al. Portosystemic encephalopathy after transjugular intrahepatic portosystemic shunt: results of a prospective controlled study. Hepatology 1994;20:46–55.

15. Somberg KA, Riegler JL, LaBerge JM, et al. Hepatic encephalopathy after transjugular intrahepatic portosystemic shunt: incidence and risk factors. Am J Gastroenterol 1995;90:549–55.

16. Riggio O, Merli M, Pedretti R, et al. Hepatic encephalopathy after transjugular intrahepatic portosystemic shunt. Incidence and risk factors. Dig Dis Sci 1996;41: 578–84.

17. Sarfeh IJ, Rypins EB. Partial versus total portacaval shunt in alcoholic cirrhosis: results of a prospective, randomized clinical trial. Ann Surg 1994;219:353–61.

18. Riggio O, Nicolao F, Angeloni S, et al. Intractable hepatic encephalopathy after TIPS with polytetrafluoroethylene-covered stent-graft. Scand J Gastroenterol 2002;37: 249–52.

19. Nolte W, Wiltfang J, Schindler C, et al. Portosystemic hepatic encephalopathy after transjugular intrahepatic portosystemic shunt in patients with cirrhosis: clinical, laboratory, psychometric, and electroencephalographic investigations. Hepatology 1998;28:1215–25.

20. Bureau C, Garcia-Pagan JC, Otal P, et al. Improved clinical outcome using polytetrafluoroethylene-coated stents for TIPS: results of a randomized study. Gastroenterology 2004;126:469–75.

21. Alvarez W, Piera C, Bandi JC, et al. Quantification of the extent of portal systemic shunting before and after TIPS: relationship with portal systemic encephalopathy. Hepatology 1995;22:296A.

22. Cabrera J, Maynar M, Granados R, et al. TIPS vs. sclerotherapy in the elective treatment of variceal hemorrhage. Gastroenterology 1996;110:832–9.

23. Zuckerman DA, Darcy MD, Bocchini TP, et al. Encephalopathy after transjugular intrahepatic portosystemic shunting: analysis and incidence of potential risk factors. AJR Am J Roentgenol 1997;169:1727–31.

24. Rossle M, Haag K, Ochs A, et al. The transjugular intrahepatic portosystemic stent-shunt procedure for variceal bleeding. N Engl J Med 1994;330:165–71.

25. Jalan R, Elton RA, Redhead DN, et al. Analysis of prognostic variables in the prediction of mortality, shunt failure, variceal rebleeding and encephalopathy following the transjugular intrahepatic portosystemic stent-shunt for variceal hemorrhage. J Hepatol 1995;23:123–8.
26. Rossle M, Deibert P, Haag K, et al. Randomised trial of transjugular-intrahepatic-portosystemic shunt versus endoscopy plus propranolol for prevention of variceal rebleeding. Lancet 1997;349:1043–9.
27. Jalan R, Forrest EH, Stanley AJ, et al. A randomized trial comparing transjugular intrahepatic portosystemic stent-shunt with variceal band ligation in the prevention of rebleeding from esophageal varices. Hepatology 1997;26:1115–22.
28. Sanyal AJ, Freedman AM, Luketic VA, et al. Transjugular intrahepatic portosystemic shunts compared with endoscopic sclerotherapy for the prevention of recurrent variceal hemorrhage. A randomized, controlled trial. Ann Intern Med 1997; 126:849–57.
29. Cello JP, Ring EJ, Olcott EW, et al. Endoscopic sclerotherapy compared with percutaneous transjugular intrahepatic portosystemic shunt after initial sclerotherapy in patients with acute variceal hemorrhage. A randomized, controlled trial. Ann Intern Med 1997;126:858–65.
30. Sauer P, Theilman L, Stremmer W, et al. Transjugular intrahepatic portosystemic stent shunt versus sclerotherapy plus propranolol for variceal rebleeding. Gastroenterology 1997;113:1623–31.
31. Merli M, Salerno F, Riggio O, et al. Transjugular intrahepatic portosystemic shunt versus endoscopic sclerotherapy for the prevention of variceal bleeding in cirrhosis: a randomized multicenter trial. Hepatology 1998;27:40–5.
32. Lebrec D, Giuily N, Hadengue A, et al. Transjugular intrahepatic portosystemic shunts: comparison with paracentesis in patients with cirrhosis and refractory ascites: a randomized trial. J Hepatol 1996;25:135–44.
33. Rössle M, Ochs A, Gülberg V, et al. A comparison of paracentesis and transjugular intrahepatic portosystemic shunting in patients with ascites. N Engl J Med 2000;342:1701–17.
34. Ginès P, Uriz J, Calahorra B, et al. Transjugular intrahepatic portosystemic shunting versus paracentesis plus albumin for refractory ascites in cirrhosis. Gastroenterology 2002;123:1839–47.
35. Sanyal AJ, Genning C, Reddy KR, et al. The North American study for the treatment of refractory ascites. Gastroenterology 2003;124:634–41.
36. Salerno F, Merli M, Riggio O, et al. Randomized controlled study of TIPS versus paracentesis plus albumin in cirrhosis with severe ascites. Hepatology 2004; 40:629–35.
37. Narahara Y, Kanazawa H, Fukuda T, et al. Transjugular intrahepatic portosystemic shunt versus paracentesis plus albumin in patients with refractory ascites who have good hepatic and renal function: a prospective randomized trial. J Gastroenterol 2011;46:78–85.
38. Burroughs AK, Vangeli M. Transjugular intrahepatic portosystemic shunt versus endoscopic therapy: randomized trials for secondary prophylaxis of variceal bleeding: an updated meta-analysis. Scand J Gastroenterol 2002;37:249–52.
39. Yang Z, Han G, Wu Q, et al. Patency and clinical outcomes of transjugular intrahepatic portosystemic shunt with polytetrafluoroethylene-covered stents versus bare stents: a meta-analysis. J Gastroenterol Hepatol 2010;25:1718–25.
40. Masson S, Mardini HA, Rose JD, et al. Hepatic encephalopathy after transjugular intrahepatic portosystemic shunt insertion: a decade of experience. QJM 2008; 101:493–501.

41. Riggio O, Angeloni S, Salvatori FM, et al. Incidence, natural history, and risk factors of hepatic encephalopathy after transjugular intrahepatic portosystemic shunt with polytetrafluoroethylene-covered stent grafts. Am J Gastroenterol 2008;103: 2738–46.
42. Riggio O, Ridola L, Lucidi C, et al. Emerging issues in the use of transjugular intrahepatic portosystemic shunt (TIPS) for management of portal hypertension: time to update the guidelines? Dig Liver Dis 2010;42:462–7.
43. Casado M, Bosch J, Garcia-Pagan JC, et al. Clinical events after TIPS: correlation with hemodynamic findings. Gastroenterology 1998;114:1296–303.
44. Bai M, Qi X, Yang Z, et al. Predictors of hepatic encephalopathy after transjugular intrahepatic portosystemic shunt in cirrhotic patients: a systematic review. J Gastroenterol Hepatol 2011;26:943–51.
45. Guevara M, Baccaro ME, Rios J, et al. Risk factors for hepatic encephalopathy in patients with cirrhosis and refractory ascites: relevance of serum sodium concentration. Liver Int 2010;30:1137–42.
46. Riggio O, Masini A, Efrati C, et al. Pharmacological prophylaxis of hepatic encephalopathy after transjugular intrahepatic portosystemic shunt: a randomized controlled study. J Hepatol 2005;42:674–9.
47. Kochar N, Tripathi D, Ireland H, et al. Transjugular intrahepatic portosystemic stent shunt (TIPSS) modification in the management of post-TIPSS refractory hepatic encephalopathy. Gut 2006;55:617–23.
48. Romero-Gomez M, Jover M, Diaz-Gomez D, et al. Phosphate-activated glutaminase activity is enhanced in brain, intestine and kidneys of rats following portacaval anastomosis. World J Gastroenterol 2006;12:2406–11.
49. Riggio O, Ridola L, Angeloni S, et al. Clinical efficacy of transjugular intrahepatic portosystemic shunt created with covered stents with different diameters: results of a randomized controlled trial. J Hepatol 2010;53:267–72.
50. Colombato LA, Spahr L, Martinet JP, et al. Haemodynamic adaptation two months after transjugular intrahepatic portosystemic shunt (TIPS) in cirrhotic patients. Gut 1996;39:600–4.
51. Merli M, Valeriano V, Funaro S, et al. Modifications of cardiac function in cirrhotic patients treated with transjugular intrahepatic portosystemic shunt (TIPS). Am J Gastroenterol 2002;97:142–8.
52. Riggio O, Ridola L, Pasquale C. Hepatic encephalopathy therapy: an overview. World J Gastrointest Pharmacol Ther 2010;6:54–63.
53. Cookson DT, Zaman Z, Gordon-Smith J, et al. Management of transjugular intrahepatic portosystemic shunt (TIPS)-associated refractory hepatic encephalopathy by shunt reduction using the parallel technique: outcomes of a retrospective case series. Cardiovasc Intervent Radiol 2011;34:92–9.
54. Fanelli F, Salvatori FM, Rabuffi P, et al. Management of refractory hepatic encephalopathy after insertion of TIPS: long-term results of shunt reduction with hourglass-shaped balloon-expandable stent-graft. AJR Am J Roentgenol 2009; 193:1696–702.
55. Chung HH, Razavi MK, Sze DY, et al. Portosystemic pressure gradient during transjugular intrahepatic portosystemic shunt with Viatorr stent graft: what is the critical low threshold to avoid medically uncontrolled low pressure gradient related complications? J Gastroenterol Hepatol 2008;23:95–101.
56. Maleux G, Heye S, Verslype C, et al. Management of transjugular intrahepatic portosystemic shunt–induced refractory hepatic encephalopathy with the parallel technique: results of a clinical follow-up study. J Vasc Interv Radiol 2007;18: 986–92.

57. Kerlan RK Jr, LaBerge JM, Baker EL, et al. Successful reversal of hepatic encephalopathy with intentional occlusion of transjugular intrahepatic portosystemic shunts. J Vasc Interv Radiol 1995;6:917–21.
58. Salerno F, Cammà C, Enea M, et al. Transjugular intrahepatic portosystemic shunt for refractory ascites: a meta-analysis of individual patient data. Gastroenterology 2007;133:825–34.
59. Garcia Pagan GC, Caca K, Bureau C, et al. Early use of TIPS in patients with cirrhosis and variceal bleeding. N Engl J Med 2010;362:2370–9.
60. Lo GH, Liang HL, Chen WC, et al. A prospective, randomized controlled trial of transjugular intrahepatic portosystemic shunt versus cyanoacrylate injection in the prevention of gastric variceal rebleeding. Endoscopy 2007;39:679–85.
61. Sauer P, Hansmann J, Richter GM, et al. Endoscopic variceal ligation plus propranolol vs. transjugular intrahepatic portosystemic stent shunt: a long-term randomized trial. Endoscopy 2002;34:690–7.
62. Gülberg V, Schepke M, Geigenberger G, et al. Transjugular intrahepatic portosystemic shunting is not superior to endoscopic variceal band ligation for prevention of variceal rebleeding in cirrhotic patients: a randomized, controlled trial. Scand J Gastroenterol 2002;37:338–43.
63. Escorsell A, Banares R, García Pagan JC, et al. TIPS versus drug therapy in preventing variceal rebleeding in advanced cirrhosis: a randomized controlled trial. Hepatology 2002;35:385–92.
64. Pomier-Layrargues G, Villeneuve P, Deschenes M, et al. Transjugular intrahepatic portosystemic shunt (TIPS) versus endoscopic variceal ligation in the prevention of variceal rebleeding in patients with cirrhosis: a randomised trial. Gut 2001;48: 390–6.
65. Garcia Villareal L, Martinez-Lagares F, Sierra A, et al. Transjugular intrahepatic portosystemic shunt versus endoscopic sclerotherapy for the prevention of variceal rebleeding after recent variceal hemorrhage. Hepatology 1999;29:27–32.

Extent of Reversibility of Hepatic Encephalopathy Following Liver Transplantation

R. Todd Frederick, MD

KEYWORDS

- Hepatic encephalopathy • Hepatocerebral degeneration
- Liver transplantation • Cerebral edema • Cerebral atrophy

Hepatic encephalopathy (HE) continues to complicate the lives of patients with cirrhosis and their caregivers. Most patients with decompensated cirrhosis awaiting liver transplantation suffer from this complication. Whether patients develop overt HE (OHE) requiring repeated hospital stays or, more commonly, minimal or covert HE with no easily recognizable signs, the burden of disease is severe.[1] Quality of life is diminished in patients with cirrhosis with HE versus those without, even if only minimal HE (MHE) is considered.[2–4] The burden of HE on caregivers is also important to consider because patients with this disorder usually cannot work or manage their own finances, cannot drive, and many cannot take care of themselves or be left alone.[5] Patients and their caregivers await their chance for liver transplantation (LT) with the expectation that all of their symptoms related to cirrhosis, including HE, will resolve. Historically, this expectation has been shared by transplant clinicians. However, recent data have revealed that this may not always be the case.

PATHOPHYSIOLOGY, NATURAL HISTORY, AND TREATMENT OF HE

The pathophysiology of HE is discussed elsewhere in this issue and can be found summarized in **Box 1** as well as in recent reviews.[6,7] The initial treatment of HE in those patients presenting with OHE usually requires removal and stabilization of any

Disclosures: The author has served as a consultant as well as a member of the Speaker's Bureau for Salix Pharmaceuticals.
Division of Hepatology, Department of Transplantation, California Pacific Medical Center, 2340 Clay Street, 3rd Floor, San Francisco, CA 94115, USA
E-mail address: fredertz@sutterhealth.org

Clin Liver Dis 16 (2012) 147–158
doi:10.1016/j.cld.2011.12.004
1089-3261/12/$ – see front matter © 2012 Elsevier Inc. All rights reserved.

> **Box 1**
> **An overview of the theories for the pathogenesis of HE.**
>
> *Toxins:*
> - Ammonia
> - Manganese
> - Byproducts of tryptophan metabolism (oxindole, indole)
> - Short-chain fatty acids
>
> *Neurologic mediators:*
> - Neurosteroids (eg, allopregnanolone)
> - Increased GABA-ergic tone
> - Endogenous benzodiazepines
> - NMDA-glutamate hyperexcitability
> - Increased acetylcholinesterase
> - False neurotransmitters (eg, octopamine)
>
> *Inflammatory mediators:*
> - TNF-a
> - IL-6
> - Reactive oxygen species
> - Reactive nitrogen species
>
> *Structural damage:*
> - Alzheimer type II astrocytosis
> - Cerebellar degeneration
> - Mammillary body and thalamic lesions
> - Globus pallidus lesions
>
> *Cerebral Edema:*
> - Hyponatremia → depletion of osmolytes
> - Ammonia → glutamine
>
> *Abbreviations:* IL, interleukin; TNF, tumor necrosis factor.

precipitating factor if one can be identified (eg, gastrointestinal bleeding, infection, psychotropic or sedating medications, electrolyte disturbance, dehydration, or constipation). Some patients do not have recurrence of HE following resolution of one of these precipitated HE events and therefore maintenance therapy is not necessary. However, most patients who have developed OHE, precipitated or spontaneous, are destined to develop recurrences; worse, many live with chronic persistent HE, ameliorated only by continuous use of medications. Treatment of OHE beyond removing or managing precipitating events entails use of nonabsorbable disaccharides such as lactulose as well as antibiotics, either systemic or poorly absorbed oral antibiotics such as rifaximin (Xifaxan). The disaccharides are used as "food" for the natural enteric flora, particularly those bacteria that produce more favorable byproducts such as Lactobacilli or Bifidobacteria.[8] In this sense, the disaccharides are prebiotics, metabolized for energy and carbons incorporated into the physical structure of the bacterium, possibly allowing these more favorable species to flourish at the expense of other enteric flora that produce more potentially noxious byproducts, such as Staphylococci or enteric gram-negative rods. Excess ammonia in the body has long been thought to arise from colonic bacterial species with urease enzyme activity, predominantly gram-negative anaerobes, Enterobacteriaceae, *Proteus*, and *Clostridium* species. The other proposed mechanisms of action of lactulose include a cathartic effect to help remove toxins such as ammonia from the gut lumen before they can be fully absorbed. The fermentation of lactulose also produces an acidic environment, thereby protonating the ammonia molecule (NH_3) to ammonium (NH_4^+), which is less able to be absorbed across the epithelial lining of the gut.

Antibiotics are commonly used in the treatment of OHE, initially in broad-spectrum intravenous form until infection has been ruled out (or treated), and then often in the oral, poorly absorbed form of rifaximin. The mechanism of action for antibiotics for treatment of HE is assumed to be related to the direct effect on bacteria, but this remains unproven. One of the suspected mechanisms is by reducing the degree of endotoxemia or translocation of bacteria into the bloodstream or ascites, which can act synergistically with ammonia or other toxins to produce OHE.[9] Alternatively, it has been proposed that the mechanism of action of neomycin, another poorly absorbed antibiotic, may be through the inhibition of intestinal glutaminase, thereby limiting the production of ammonia from glutamine.[10]

REVERSIBILITY OF HE: THE CONCEPT

Traditionally, it has been proposed that most OHE events are at least potentially reversible, with only those patients succumbing to the precipitating event (ie, bleeding, infection) not manifesting reversibility. If patients are able to regain consciousness and survive a severe HE event, they typically seem to return to their baseline level of cognitive functioning with supportive care,[11] or with disaccharides,[12] or with rifaximin.[13] A subset of patients with OHE continue to suffer from symptoms and are classified as chronic persistent HE that may not be reversible with medical therapy.[14]

Low-grade cerebral edema is now thought to explain at least part of the pathophysiology of HE in cirrhosis and would in theory be reversible with successful medical therapy or following LT.[15,16] However, neuropathologic characteristics are found in the brains of patients with HE at autopsy, suggesting that the concept of complete reversibility requires more in-depth analysis.

REVERSIBILITY OF HE: MEDICAL TREATMENT

Most clinicians attest that the reversibility of OHE following resolution of the precipitating event and management of hyperammonemia is the norm rather than the exception. However, considering the full spectrum of HE from overt to minimal, one must further scrutinize whether patients with OHE episodes truly return to normal cognitive functioning. The questions can be raised, "Do patients with episodes of OHE return to their previous level of functioning or is there an irreversible component? If so, is there cumulative damage after repeated episodes of HE?" Recently investigators seem to have answered these questions.[17,18] In one study,[17] investigators analyzed the cognitive function of 226 cirrhotic patients (54 prior OHE, 120 MHE, 52 no HE) using standard psychometric testing and the inhibitory control test (ICT). Those patients with prior OHE episodes scored statistically lower than those without prior OHE, and, even compared with patients with MHE, they showed significant deficiencies in learning on the ICT. Followed prospectively, those patients subsequently experiencing OHE developed significant abnormalities on follow-up psychometric testing that did not manifest in those cirrhotic patients without OHE episodes. Most alarmingly, these deficiencies were directly correlated with the number of admissions for OHE, suggesting that each episode of OHE contributed to the patient's subsequent cognitive decline. Despite treatment intended to lower ammonia, these deficits persisted. Radiologic and autopsy data were not available in this study. The investigators postulate that toxins other than ammonia, such as manganese, inflammatory cytokines, or mercaptans, may be implicated in this persistent cognitive dysfunction. These additional toxic insults would hopefully be reversed with other medical therapy or with LT.

In another recent study,[18] investigators used the more validated psychometric hepatic encephalopathy score (PHES), administered on 2 occasions 3 days apart to 106 cirrhotic patients (27 prior OHE, 34 MHE, 45 no HE), to determine whether a learning effect could be shown. Patients with prior OHE were less likely to show any learning effect during the second PHES testing compared with patients without HE or those with MHE. Even the 8 patients with prior OHE but with baseline normal PHES (ie, no residual MHE) failed to show a learning effect, whereas the patients with no MHE (normal PHES) and no prior OHE were able to improve their PHES on the second assessment 3 days later, showing intact learning ability. The investigators concluded that patients do not fully recover following an episode of OHE.

Perhaps patients with OHE episodes then remain in a state of MHE following the OHE event, thereby explaining their impaired performances on psychometric testing. However, this does not entirely explain the spectrum of deficits seen in this disease because many patients with MHE have never experienced OHE, although they are known to be at increased risk.[19] Conversely, not all patients who develop an episode of OHE are subsequently categorized as impaired on follow-up psychometric testing. In addition, it seems that treatment of MHE can improve the neurocognitive deficits of this disorder,[20,21] whereas the deficits after OHE did not seem to ameliorate with treatment.[17] Perhaps the episodes of OHE create incremental structural or histologic damage in the cirrhotic patient's brain that is not reversible with medical treatment.

This concept is not new, and was first reported in 1914 by the French physician van Woerkom.[22] In the 1960s it was termed acquired hepatocerebral degeneration (AHCD), to be distinguished from familial or wilsonian hepatolenticular degeneration, with which it was found to be similar on neuropathology.[23,24] Victor and colleagues,[24] while studying hepatic coma in the late 1940s noted that, "survivors of this condition occasionally manifested a relatively permanent disorder of nervous function." There was no specific therapy (eg, lactulose, antibiotics) for this altered neurologic function at that time, and what was once considered permanent may now be reversible with more modern medical care.

A similar but distinct syndrome of hepatic myelopathy (HM) also involves chronic persistent neurologic dysfunction, primarily manifesting as rigidity, paraparesis or tetraparesis, and/or parkinsonism without prominent cognitive dysfunction. One important feature common to both AHCD and HM is the presence of large portosystemic shunts, either spontaneous or surgically placed. These disorders have also been described in patients with spontaneous or surgical shunts without intrinsic liver disease, analogous to type B HE. Whether AHCD and HM should be considered as part of the spectrum of HE or as distinct entities remains unanswered. AHCD seems to be difficult to discern clinically from that of chronic persistent HE, which is also associated with a high prevalence of portosystemic shunts.[25] AHCD seems to be associated with a more prominent motor dysfunction, often with extrapyramidal signs, ataxia, craniofacial dyskinesias, choreoathetosis, or dysarthria; whereas cognitive dysfunction may or may not be problematic.[26] Many patients with AHCD and/or HM have suffered from repeated episodes of hepatic coma and it seems likely that these syndromes are a consequence of these OHE events, rather than unrelated entities. More recent series of cirrhotic patients have estimated that AHCD and HM are rare in this population, at roughly 0.8% to 2% of cases,[27,28] although this may be an under-estimation caused by lack of recognition of the syndrome.[29] Little can be found in the hepatology literature regarding AHCD and HM, and they likely remain grossly under-diagnosed by gastroenterologists and hepatologists because of lack of recognition.

The distinctive pathologic findings of AHCD involve not only the reactive Alzheimer type II gliosis commonly found in the brains of cirrhotic patients with HE but also gray matter spongiform or polymicrocavitation changes and generalized cerebral atrophy. One theory has asserted that manganese deposition within the basal ganglia also plays a prominent role in these disorders and is thought to represent the T1 hyperintensity of the globus pallidus on magnetic resonance imaging (MRI) commonly seen in patients with AHCD. Such structural damage has been identified in the brains of cirrhotic patients on autopsy,[30–33] as well as in imaging studies[34]; however, direct correlates to implicate the cause of these defects have not been proven. Treatment of AHCD and HM is limited. Options such as ammonia-lowering medications (disaccharides), antibiotics, levodopa, anticholinergics, and manganese chelators (eg, ethylenediaminepentaacetic acid [EDTA]) have been tried with minimal success, which prompts the question of whether this documented neurologic disorder is possibly reversible with LT or do these patients suffer from a progressive neurodegenerative disease?

REVERSIBILITY OF HE: LIVER TRANSPLANTATION

With successful LT, the problems of synthetic and excretory dysfunction of the failing liver are restored to normal. In addition, the portal hypertension and portosystemic shunting are also improved, if not entirely resolved. Therefore, it would be expected that the symptoms of OHE, as well as the abnormal psychometric testing in patients with MHE, would completely resolve after LT. However, not all post-LT patients have completely intact neurocognitive functioning, especially when highly sensitive testing methods are used. In this scenario, it is important to consider all of the possible causes of post-LT neurologic dysfunction, of which HE is only 1 (**Box 2**), before concluding that HE is not reversible.

Most patients with OHE have resolution of their symptoms following successful LT, with few exceptions, although it may take several weeks before the sensorium fully clears.[35] However, when specialized testing is performed, many of these patients are recognized as having persistent structural abnormalities of the brain or are cognitively impaired. The methods of testing have included MRI, magnetic resonance spectroscopy (MRS), positron emission tomography (PET) scanning, psychometric or computerized testing, or electroencephalography (EEG).

Several investigators using MRI and MRS[15,36–39] or PET of the brain[40] have shown resolution of the radiologic correlates of HE following LT, whereas others have come to different conclusions.[41,42] The normalization of the MRS changes reflects a rebalancing of neuronal and astrocyte intracellular osmoles and amino acids, (eg, myoinositol, glutamine) and may take several months to manifest,[43] but tends to precede the resolution of the T1 hyperintensity within the globus pallidus. MRS normalization correlated better with the timing of improved psychometric testing.[36] It seems that the MRI T1 hyperintensity of the globus pallidus takes longer to reverse and was noted to resolve after 12 months in one study[36] and after 10 to 12 months in another study,[38] but correlated poorly with resolution of MHE. The improvement in MRS likely represents reversal of low-grade cerebral edema in the cirrhotic brain,[15] whereas the T1

Box 2
Potential causes of post-LT neurologic dysfunction

Liver or transplant related:

- Residual HE
  - Persistent hyperammonemia or other toxins
  - Irreversible neurologic injury from prior overt HE
    - AHCD
    - Hepatic myelopathy
    - Cirrhotic parkinsonism
- Residual portosystemic shunting
- Medication side effects: calcineurin inhibitors, steroids, anticonvulsants, opiates, sleeping aids
  - Posterior reversible encephalopathy syndrome (particularly with cyclosporine)
- Ischemic brain injury related to hypoperfusion during transplantation
- Ischemic brain injury related to cerebral edema during surgery
- Rapidly corrected hyponatremia leading to central pontine myelinolysis
- Preexisting Wilson disease

Non–transplant related:

- Organic brain syndrome or traumatic brain injury
- Wernicke-Korsakoff syndrome or alcohol-induced dementia or cerebellar degeneration
- Other causes of dementia (eg, Alzheimer, multi-infarct, Parkinson, Lewy body, Pick disease, Huntington disease, multiple sclerosis)
- Seizure disorder
- Cerebrovascular accident
- Normal-pressure hydrocephalus
- Vitamin B12, folate, or niacin deficiency
- Central nervous system malignancy
- Chronic subdural hematoma
- Sepsis
- Other infections: neurosyphilis, Lyme, HIV, Cryptococcus, CMV, PML, Whipple, CJD
- Thyroid disease
- Vasculitis
- Sarcoidosis
- Porphyria

Abbreviations: CJD, Creutzfeldt-Jakob disease; CMV, Cytomegalovirus; HIV, human immunodeficiency virus; PML, progressive multifocal leukoencephalopathy.

---

hyperintensities within the basal ganglia likely represent manganese deposition and correlate with degree of liver insufficiency and with the presence of parkinsonian disturbances in cirrhotic patients.[44] Most recently, investigators have used voxel-based morphometry MRI of the brains of cirrhotic patients as a means of assessing brain tissue density.[42] This technique has been found to correlate with brain atrophy in neurodegenerative diseases such as Huntington and Alzheimer. The study included 48 cirrhotic patients (17 prior OHE, 18 with MHE) and 51 healthy controls. In addition, 12 patients were studied a median 11 months after LT. The gray and white matter densities of the brains of cirrhotic patients were significantly decreased compared with controls. There were linear progressions in decreased brain density from Childs class A to C as well as in patients without HE versus MHE versus with prior OHE. Of the 12 patients with post-LT imaging, the findings of decreased brain density were noted to persist compared with controls. Psychometric testing for possible residual cognitive deficits were not performed in this group. The investigators concluded that patients with advancing cirrhosis and with HE experience decreasing density of the brain that likely correlates with progressive neuronal cell loss akin to other neurodegenerative diseases, and these changes do not seem to reverse with LT.

Psychometric testing is increasingly used to detect changes of MHE and has been studied in the posttransplant setting. For patients with MHE before LT, investigators have found conflicting results regarding its resolution following LT. In the first study to assess reversibility of MHE following transplantation, Tarter and colleagues[45] examined 62 patients with cirrhosis without OHE awaiting transplantation and compared them with healthy controls, as well as patients with Crohn disease, chosen to control for medical illness, immunosuppressive drug therapy, and the effect of the longitudinal physician-patient relationship. They were given a battery of 27 psychometric tests before transplantation and then retested a mean of 60 weeks after LT. The cirrhotic patients performed poorly on 12 of the 27 tests before LT compared with healthy controls, but on only 4 of 27 when compared with patients with Crohn disease, suggesting that at least some of the deficit was related to chronic illness in general, rather than MHE. In follow-up testing, the post-LT patients showed significant improvements but still underperformed on 4 of 27 tests, particularly those measuring attentional and psychomotor capacities. The investigators concluded that MHE improves, but may not entirely reverse, after LT, and perhaps a permanent neurologic abnormality develops following years of chronic liver disease. A valid alternative hypothesis was also raised regarding the effects of immunosuppression, particularly cyclosporine, on psychomotor performance. Information regarding neuroimaging or extent of pre-LT OHE was not provided. In another large prospective study, 78 patients without OHE undergoing evaluation for LT had psychometric testing and were compared with controls. Of these, 23 were successfully transplanted and able to undergo repeat testing 6 months after LT, whereas 13 also underwent testing at 18 months. MHE was considered resolved in all patients with significant improvements noted in most tests in both domains of attention and memory. Improvement continued to 18 months for both selective attention and verbal short-term memory and there were no differences in performance compared with controls except in memory span.[46] Another small study of 14 patients with MHE (but without significant cerebral atrophy) found that, although the mean score on a battery of psychometric tests improved following LT (a mean of 21 months after LT), they remained abnormal compared with healthy controls.[47] On further inspection, half of the patients significantly improved to the point of being considered normal, whereas the other half not only failed to improve but worsened on repeat testing after LT. This group had particular difficulty with visuomotor deficits. None of the clinical or demographic factors analyzed by the investigators (cause of cirrhosis, age, education, severity or duration of liver disease, extent of OHE, type of immunosuppression, history of gastrointestinal bleeding, or presence of esophageal varices) helped to predict which patients may not improve after LT. Neuroimaging was performed to exclude patients with severe atrophy, but follow-up imaging was not reported. The most recent study to analyze post-LT cognitive dysfunction combined a neuropsychological assessment before and after LT with brain MRI and MRS findings.[48] These investigators enrolled 70 consecutive cirrhotic patients awaiting LT (24 with prior OHE, 28 with MHE) and administered the neuropsychological testing 2 months before LT and 6 to 12 months after in 52 of them. Twenty-four of these patients also underwent brain MRI and MRS. There was significant improvement on follow-up testing; however, 7 patients (13%) did not show improvement and remained mildly impaired. These patients had higher rates of alcoholic liver disease, more diabetes, and more episodes of OHE (71%) than those without residual impairment (OHE in 42%). Those with prior OHE primarily showed deficiencies in motor function. MRI showed more brain atrophy in patients with OHE and this correlated directly with duration of HE. The investigators concluded that OHE has a detrimental effect on post-LT cognition, likely related to cerebral atrophy. Repeated episodes of OHE and an extended duration between the first OHE episode and the time of LT may lead to permanent neuronal cell loss.

With knowledge of the neuropathologic correlates of AHCD and HM, these disorders, unlike HE, might not be expected to improve following LT. Interestingly, although data are conflicting in this regard, it seems that most patients undergoing LT with these syndromes do show significant improvement, typically within the first few months.[27,49–51] However, other investigators have shown a lack of complete resolution of some motor disorders such as parkinsonism after LT, although with only limited follow-up.[41] These patients continued to show pallidal T1 hyperintensity at 4 months after LT, but other studies show that these densities may take up to a year to reverse.[36,38]

As mentioned earlier and as outlined in **Box 2**, there are many potential reasons for patients to have persistent or de novo neurologic dysfunction following LT. It has been estimated that 10% to 25% of patients undergoing LT suffer from neurologic complications such as metabolic encephalopathy or seizures, typically within the first month.[35] Patients with OHE at the time of LT seem to have a tenfold risk of postoperative neurologic complications.[35] Persistence of portosystemic shunting has been reported after LT and may contribute to persistent neurologic deficits including HE[52,53] as well as AHCD.[28] Patients undergoing LT often face massive volume fluctuations related to clamping and release of major vessels and blood loss, triggering extreme fluxes in blood pressure, electrolyte concentrations, acid-base status, and perfusion pressures. Studies of cerebral oxygen consumption during LT have shown significantly reduced cerebral metabolism in patients with OHE that rapidly corrected following reperfusion of the graft, suggesting that these patients may be at higher risk of additional neurologic compromise as a result of this surgery.[54]

To fully assess the relationship and implications of OHE, MHE, or AHCD with post-LT cognitive dysfunction, the effect on quality of life (QoL) of the LT recipient must be analyzed. Both MHE and OHE negatively affect QoL in patients with cirrhosis.[4] Tarter and colleagues[55] found that more advanced HE before LT predicted less improvement in QoL after LT compared with patients without significant neurologic impairment as measured by the sickness impact profile. Lewis and Howdle[56] followed a small group of patients for 10 or more years after LT and found a significant correlation between residual cognitive dysfunction and reduced QoL, as expected. A large study of 164 patients with end-stage liver disease followed prospectively for 3 years found significant improvements in both QoL and cognitive function in the LT recipients despite an increased baseline prevalence of memory impairment, psychomotor slowing, anxiety, and depression in this group. Severity of pre-LT liver disease did not predict any decrement in QoL after LT.[57]

SUMMARY

The evidence suggests that HE is not completely reversible, even with LT. A novel concept of reversible delirium-like and irreversible dementia-like components of HE has been proposed in an effort to better understand this problem.[58] The reversible components are likely related to the low-grade cerebral edema triggered by astrocyte swelling from ammonia and glutamine influx and compensated for by myoinositol efflux. Basal ganglia hyperintensity, which tends to correlate with the psychomotor dysfunction of HE, seems to resolve more slowly but is reversible. In addition, the more pathologic changes of neuronal cell loss, microcavitation, and cerebral atrophy associated with prolonged periods of both OHE and MHE seem to represent the more irreversible dementia-like or neurodegenerative component of HE. However, despite this sobering finding of permanent cognitive dysfunction despite lifesaving LT, it is reassuring to note that most patients undergoing LT do not develop irreversible MHE. Future research should focus on methods of identifying the minority of patients who will develop permanent neurocognitive dysfunction and assessing means of neuroprevention.

REFERENCES

1. Poordad FF. Review article: the burden of hepatic encephalopathy. Aliment Pharmacol Ther 2007;25(Suppl 1):3–9.
2. Amodio P. Health related quality of life and minimal hepatic encephalopathy. It is time to insert 'quality' in health care. J Gastroenterol Hepatol 2009;24(3):329–30.
3. Bao ZJ, Qiu DK, Ma X, et al. Assessment of health-related quality of life in Chinese patients with minimal hepatic encephalopathy. World J Gastroenterol 2007;13(21):3003–8.
4. Arguedas MR, DeLawrence TG, McGuire BM. Influence of hepatic encephalopathy on health-related quality of life in patients with cirrhosis. Dig Dis Sci 2003; 48(8):1622–6.
5. Bajaj JS, Wade JB, Gibson DP, et al. The multi-dimensional burden of cirrhosis and hepatic encephalopathy on patients and caregivers. Am J Gastroenterol 2011;106(9):1646–53.
6. Frederick RT. Current concepts in the pathophysiology and management of hepatic encephalopathy. Gastroenterol Hepatol (N Y) 2011;7(4):222–33.
7. Prakash R, Mullen KD. Mechanisms, diagnosis and management of hepatic encephalopathy. Nat Rev Gastroenterol Hepatol 2010;7(9):515–25.
8. Conn HO, Floch MH. Effects of lactulose and Lactobacillus acidophilus on the fecal flora. Am J Clin Nutr 1970;23(12):1588–94.
9. Blei AT. Infection, inflammation and hepatic encephalopathy, synergism redefined. J Hepatol 2004;40(2):327–30.
10. Hawkins RA, Jessy J, Mans AM, et al. Neomycin reduces the intestinal production of ammonia from glutamine. Adv Exp Med Biol 1994;368:125–34.
11. Jalan R, Kapoor D. Reversal of diuretic-induced hepatic encephalopathy with infusion of albumin but not colloid. Clin Sci (Lond) 2004;106(5):467–74.
12. Elkington SG, Floch MH, Conn HO. Lactulose in the treatment of chronic portal-systemic encephalopathy. A double-blind clinical trial. N Engl J Med 1969;281(8): 408–12.
13. Mas A, Rodés J, Sunyer L, et al. Comparison of rifaximin and lactitol in the treatment of acute hepatic encephalopathy: results of a randomized, double-blind, double-dummy, controlled clinical trial. J Hepatol 2003;38(1):51–8.
14. Ferenci P, Lockwood A, Mullen K, et al. Hepatic encephalopathy–definition, nomenclature, diagnosis, and quantification: final report of the working party at

the 11th World Congresses of Gastroenterology, Vienna, 1998. Hepatology 2002; 35(3):716–21.

15. Cordoba J, Alonso J, Rovira A, et al. The development of low-grade cerebral edema in cirrhosis is supported by the evolution of (1)H-magnetic resonance abnormalities after liver transplantation. J Hepatol 2001;35(5):598–604.

16. Haussinger D. Low grade cerebral edema and the pathogenesis of hepatic encephalopathy in cirrhosis. Hepatology 2006;43(6):1187–90.

17. Bajaj JS, Schubert CM, Heuman DM, et al. Persistence of cognitive impairment after resolution of overt hepatic encephalopathy. Gastroenterology 2010;138(7): 2332–40.

18. Riggio O, Ridola L, Pasquale C, et al. Evidence of persistent cognitive impairment after resolution of overt hepatic encephalopathy. Clin Gastroenterol Hepatol 2011; 9(2):181–3.

19. Bajaj JS, Saeian K, Verber MD, et al. Inhibitory control test is a simple method to diagnose minimal hepatic encephalopathy and predict development of overt hepatic encephalopathy. Am J Gastroenterol 2007;102(4):754–60.

20. Bajaj JS, Heuman DM, Wade JB, et al. Rifaximin improves driving simulator performance in a randomized trial of patients with minimal hepatic encephalopathy. Gastroenterology 2011;140(2):478–87.e1.

21. Prasad S, Dhiman RK, Duseja A, et al. Lactulose improves cognitive functions and health-related quality of life in patients with cirrhosis who have minimal hepatic encephalopathy. Hepatology 2007;45(3):549–59.

22. van Woerkom W. La cirrhose hepatique avec alterations dans les centres nerveux evoluant chez des sujets d'age moyen. Nouvelle iconographie de la Salpetriere 1914;7:41 [In French].

23. Meissner W, Tison F. Acquired hepatocerebral degeneration. Handb Clin Neurol 2011;100:193–7.

24. Victor M, Adams RD, Cole M. The acquired (non-Wilsonian) type of chronic hepatocerebral degeneration. Medicine (Baltimore) 1965;44(5):345–96.

25. Riggio O, Efrati C, Catalano C, et al. High prevalence of spontaneous portal-systemic shunts in persistent hepatic encephalopathy: a case-control study. Hepatology 2005;42(5):1158–65.

26. Ferrara J, Jankovic J. Acquired hepatocerebral degeneration. J Neurol 2009; 256(3):320–32.

27. Pinarbasi B, Kaymakoglu S, Matur Z, et al. Are acquired hepatocerebral degeneration and hepatic myelopathy reversible? J Clin Gastroenterol 2009;43(2): 176–81.

28. Fernández-Rodriguez R, Contreras A, De Villoria JG, et al. Acquired hepatocerebral degeneration: clinical characteristics and MRI findings. Eur J Neurol 2010; 17(12):1463–70.

29. Burkhard PR, Delavelle J, Du Pasquier R, et al. Chronic parkinsonism associated with cirrhosis: a distinct subset of acquired hepatocerebral degeneration. Arch Neurol 2003;60(4):521–8.

30. Bergeron M, Reader TA, Layrargues GP, et al. Monoamines and metabolites in autopsied brain tissue from cirrhotic patients with hepatic encephalopathy. Neurochem Res 1989;14(9):853–9.

31. Kril JJ, Butterworth RF. Diencephalic and cerebellar pathology in alcoholic and nonalcoholic patients with end-stage liver disease. Hepatology 1997;26(4): 837–41.

32. Butterworth RF. Neuronal cell death in hepatic encephalopathy. Metab Brain Dis 2007;22(3–4):309–20.

33. Matsusue E, Kinoshita T, Ohama E, et al. Cerebral cortical and white matter lesions in chronic hepatic encephalopathy: MR-pathologic correlations. AJNR Am J Neuroradiol 2005;26(2):347–51.
34. Krieger S, Jauss M, Jansen O, et al. Neuropsychiatric profile and hyperintense globus pallidus on T1-weighted magnetic resonance images in liver cirrhosis. Gastroenterology 1996;111(1):147–55.
35. Dhar R, Young GB, Marotta P. Perioperative neurological complications after liver transplantation are best predicted by pre-transplant hepatic encephalopathy. Neurocrit Care 2008;8(2):253–8.
36. Naegele T, Grodd W, Viebahn R, et al. MR imaging and (1)H spectroscopy of brain metabolites in hepatic encephalopathy: time-course of renormalization after liver transplantation. Radiology 2000;216(3):683–91.
37. Rovira A, Mínguez B, Aymerich FX, et al. Decreased white matter lesion volume and improved cognitive function after liver transplantation. Hepatology 2007; 46(5):1485–90.
38. Pujol A, Pujol J, Graus F, et al. Hyperintense globus pallidus on T1-weighted MRI in cirrhotic patients is associated with severity of liver failure. Neurology 1993; 43(1):65–9.
39. Weissenborn K, Ehrenheim C, Hori A, et al. Pallidal lesions in patients with liver cirrhosis: clinical and MRI evaluation. Metab Brain Dis 1995;10(3):219–31.
40. Burra P, Dam M, Chierichetti F, et al. 18F-fluorodeoxyglucose positron emission tomography study of brain metabolism in cirrhosis: effect of liver transplantation. Transplant Proc 1999;31(1–2):418–20.
41. Lazeyras F, Spahr L, DuPasquier R, et al. Persistence of mild parkinsonism 4 months after liver transplantation in patients with preoperative minimal hepatic encephalopathy: a study on neuroradiological and blood manganese changes. Transpl Int 2002;15(4):188–95.
42. Guevara M, Baccaro ME, Gómez-Ansón B, et al. Cerebral magnetic resonance imaging reveals marked abnormalities of brain tissue density in patients with cirrhosis without overt hepatic encephalopathy. J Hepatol 2011;55(3): 564–73.
43. Huda A, Guze BH, Thomas A, et al. Clinical correlation of neuropsychological tests with 1H magnetic resonance spectroscopy in hepatic encephalopathy. Psychosom Med 1998;60(5):550–6.
44. Spahr L, Vingerhoets F, Lazeyras F, et al. Magnetic resonance imaging and proton spectroscopic alterations correlate with parkinsonian signs in patients with cirrhosis. Gastroenterology 2000;119(3):774–81.
45. Tarter RE, Switala JA, Arria A, et al. Subclinical hepatic encephalopathy. Comparison before and after orthotopic liver transplantation. Transplantation 1990;50(4): 632–7.
46. Mattarozzi K, Stracciari A, Vignatelli L, et al. Minimal hepatic encephalopathy: longitudinal effects of liver transplantation. Arch Neurol 2004;61(2):242–7.
47. Mechtcheriakov S, Graziadei IW, Mattedi M, et al. Incomplete improvement of visuo-motor deficits in patients with minimal hepatic encephalopathy after liver transplantation. Liver Transpl 2004;10(1):77–83.
48. Garcia-Martinez R, Rovira A, Alonso J, et al. Hepatic encephalopathy is associated with posttransplant cognitive function and brain volume. Liver Transpl 2011;17(1):38–46.
49. Powell EE, Pender MP, Chalk JB, et al. Improvement in chronic hepatocerebral degeneration following liver transplantation. Gastroenterology 1990;98(4): 1079–82.

50. Weissenborn K, Tietge UJ, Bokemeyer M, et al. Liver transplantation improves hepatic myelopathy: evidence by three cases. Gastroenterology 2003;124(2): 346–51.
51. Stracciari A, Guarino M, Pazzaglia P, et al. Acquired hepatocerebral degeneration: full recovery after liver transplantation. J Neurol Neurosurg Psychiatry 2001;70(1):136–7.
52. Braun MM, Bar-Nathan N, Shaharabani E, et al. Postshunt hepatic encephalopathy in liver transplant recipients. Transplantation 2009;87(5):734–9.
53. Herrero JI, Bilbao JI, Diaz ML, et al. Hepatic encephalopathy after liver transplantation in a patient with a normally functioning graft: treatment with embolization of portosystemic collaterals. Liver Transpl 2009;15(1):111–4.
54. Philips BJ, Armstrong IR, Pollock A, et al. Cerebral blood flow and metabolism in patients with chronic liver disease undergoing orthotopic liver transplantation. Hepatology 1998;27(2):369–76.
55. Tarter RE, Switala J, Plail J, et al. Severity of hepatic encephalopathy before liver transplantation is associated with quality of life after transplantation. Arch Intern Med 1992;152(10):2097–101.
56. Lewis MB, Howdle PD. Cognitive dysfunction and health-related quality of life in long-term liver transplant survivors. Liver Transpl 2003;9(11):1145–8.
57. O'Carroll RE, Couston M, Cossar J, et al. Psychological outcome and quality of life following liver transplantation: a prospective, national, single-center study. Liver Transpl 2003;9(7):712–20.
58. Rose C, Jalan R. Is minimal hepatic encephalopathy completely reversible following liver transplantation? Liver Transpl 2004;10(1):84–7.

Hepatic Encephalopathy and Health-Related Quality of Life

Giampaolo Bianchi, MD, Marco Giovagnoli, MD,
Anna Simona Sasdelli, MD, Giulio Marchesini, MD*

KEYWORDS

- Health status • Hepatic encephalopathy • Liver cirrhosis
- Depression

In past decades there has been a growing interest in the medical literature on patients' quality of life (QoL). QoL is a broad and multidimensional concept, without a universally shared definition. The World Health Organization defines QoL as "the individuals' perception of their position in life in the context of the culture and value system in which they live and in relation to their goals, standards, and concerns."[1] In other words, QoL includes all aspects of human well-being, physical and cognitive skills, social functioning, set of emotions, and psychological status.

Because of this wide definition, QoL depends on a variety of psychosocial factors, including relations, income, occupation, and health, and a comprehensive assessment cannot be obtained on a subjective basis. More feasible is a limited assessment in relation to specific problems, such as health status. Health-related quality of life (HRQoL) thus indicates the subjective perception of QoL in relation to acute and chronic diseases, limiting patients' positions within their social context, based on 3 major components: physical functioning (eg, strength or weakness), psychological functioning (mood and emotional status), and social functioning (public relations, work).[2]

The patients' perspectives of their health status, as previously defined, has gained a central role in the measurement of medical interventions and disease outcomes. Most patients believe that HRQoL is more important than longevity; in several circumstances they are much more interested in quality and disability prevention than in survival. Consequently, the goal of medical interventions becomes the prevention and treatment of symptoms and complications and the maintenance of patients'

The authors have no conflicts of interest to disclose.
Department of Medicine and Surgery, S. Orsola-Malpighi Hospital, "Alma Mater Studiorum" University of Bologna, Via Massarenti 9, 40138 Bologna, Italy
* Corresponding author.
E-mail address: giulio.marchesini@unibo.it

Clin Liver Dis 16 (2012) 159–170
doi:10.1016/j.cld.2011.12.003
1089-3261/12/$ – see front matter © 2012 Elsevier Inc. All rights reserved.

social functioning, not solely the prevention of death.[3] Most regulatory agencies now consider that a subjective measure of patients' health status may be included, together with objective parameters, such as biochemical values or survival rate, in the evaluation of cost-benefit ratio of medical and surgical interventions.[4]

THE MEASUREMENT OF HRQoL

The measurement of HRQoL, however feasible, remains a difficult task, and physicians cannot rely on their personal judgment. The measurement of patients' perspectives on health status is thus based on self-administered and standardized questionnaires. Two types of questionnaires have been developed: generic and disease-specific questionnaires.[5] Generic questionnaires are widespread and easy to complete; they explore several areas considered of primary interest in relation to health, allowing a comparison between a normative control population and diseased patients or between different types of diseased populations. By definition, these instruments are scarcely sensitive; they cannot identify disease-specific alterations and slight but clinically important changes could remain undetected. For this purpose, disease-specific questionnaires have been developed to provide more specific and sensitive instruments to be used for longitudinal clinical studies.[6,7]

The most commonly used generic questionnaires for the assessment of HRQoL are the Sickness Impact Profile (SIP), the Nottingham Health Profile (NHP), and Medical Outcomes Study Short Form-36 (SF-36) (**Table 1**).[8] The SIP[9] consists of 136 items, covering 12 domains: it requires several minutes to complete and people with cognitive dysfunctions (such as those with metabolic encephalopathy) could fail to complete the questionnaire. The NHP[10] has been developed to measure distress and is especially useful in more severe levels of disability, but is less sensitive to mild changes.[11] The SF-36[12] is applicable in a wide variety of pathologic conditions, from subjects with severe disability to the general population.[13] It is easy to complete and has a good sensitivity, which makes the SF-36 the best and most frequently used instrument in clinical practice.

Specific questionnaires have been developed for a variety of chronic diseases, such as renal and cardiac failure, liver cirrhosis, diabetes, and osteoarticular diseases, which have a great impact on patients' HRQoL. Probably the most widely used

Table 1
Generic instruments in the assessment of health-related quality of life

Sickness Impact Profile	Nottingham Health Profile	Medical Outcome Survey Short-Form 36
1. Sleep and rest	Part I—present distress	1. Physical functioning
2. Eating	1. Energy	2. Role limitation—
3. Work	2. Sleep	physical
4. Home management	3. Pain	3. Bodily pain
5. Recreation and pastimes	4. Emotional reactions	4. General health
6. Ambulation	5. Social isolation	5. Role limitation—
7. Mobility	6. Physical mobility	emotional
8. Body care and movement	Part II—everyday activities	6. Vitality
9. Social interactions	Occupation, jobs around	7. Mental health
10. Alertness behavior	the home, social life,	8. Social functioning
11. Emotional behavior	home life, sex life,	Physical component
12. Communication	hobbies, and holidays.	summary (1–4)
Physical subscore (6–8)		Mental component
Psychosocial subscore (9–11)		summary (5–8)

specific questionnaire for assessing patients' perceived health status in chronic liver diseases is the Chronic Liver Disease Questionnaire (CLDQ),[14] a practical tool of only 29 items, which explores 6 domains frequently altered in the presence of liver dysfunction: fatigue, activity, emotional function, abdominal symptoms, systemic symptoms, and worries. The CLDQ is a feasible questionnaire also for patients affected by mild hepatic encephalopathy (HE), but its sensitivity decreases with the worsening of liver disease.

Finally, the aging of the population implies a higher prevalence of chronic illnesses, which have a great impact on daily life and a relevant social and economic burden. A good example is liver cirrhosis, because of its high prevalence in Western countries, relevant morbidity and mortality, and extremely variable clinical manifestations. Many factors may adversely affect HRQoL in patients with cirrhosis: symptoms (itching, fatigue, muscle cramps), therapeutic interventions (treatment with loop diuretics, interferon), complications (ascites, variceal bleeding, infections, encephalopathy), and restriction in social and work activities.[15,16]

HEPATIC ENCEPHALOPATHY AND HRQoL

HE is a major complication of liver cirrhosis and up to 50% of patients with cirrhosis experience a variable degree of this condition at least once in their lives.[16] Patients with HE suffer from various degrees of altered consciousness, personality changes, impaired intellectual functioning, and neuromuscular dysfunction. This complication is not immediately life threatening, but its impact on patients' functioning, social interaction, and sense of well-being is of paramount importance.[17] The occurrence of HE is, however, associated with a variety of clinical complications, which may all adversely affect HRQoL, and it is not easy to dissect the independent effect of HE on perceived health status.

Several studies showed that chronic liver diseases and cirrhosis have a negative impact on HRQoL,[18] but only a few investigated if and how much HE may negatively affect patients' perceived health status (**Table 2**). The problem is that as long as HE worsens, patients are unaware of their disease (anosognosia), as also happens in several metabolic and vascular cerebral disorders.[19] Alterations in patients' behavior and abilities are more easily recognized by people living with the patients, not by patients themselves.

Although there is a general consensus about the direct and profound impact that HE has on HRQoL,[17] this relationship cannot be evaluated during an acute episode of overt HE, because the impairment of consciousness makes the patient unable to complete the questionnaires. In 160 patients with cirrhosis attending for liver transplant evaluation, HRQoL was found to be impaired in relation to HE, but irrespective of the Child-Pugh score.[17] Using the SF-36, HE was found to have a strong impact on the mental dimension of HRQoL, whereas the severity of liver disease mainly affected the physical components. Moreover, overt HE negatively affected both physical and mental aspects, whereas subclinical encephalopathy had a significant impact on the mental health and role-emotional domains, resulting in lower scores compared with patients without encephalopathy. On the basis of these findings, the investigators suggested that all patients with cirrhosis should be screened for early detection and treatment of HE, to improve patients' HRQoL.[17]

In 554 patients with cirrhosis, evaluated either as outpatients or during hospital admission, where the SF-36 and NHP inventories were systematically applied in the absence of major signs of decompensation, the presence of HE measured by psychometric testing was associated with a poorer perceived health status in nearly all

Table 2
Principal studies on the association of hepatic encephalopathy (HE) or minimal hepatic encephalopathy (MHE) with health-related quality of life

Author, Year (Ref)	No. of Cases	Type of HE	Test	Results	Limitations
Groeneweg et al,[29] 1998 & Groeneweg et al,[30] 2000	179	MHE	SIP	Low SIP scores, mainly in alertness, sleep and rest, fine motor skills and work, are strictly linked to the presence of MHE,	The diagnostic criteria for MHE used in the survey could lead to an overestimation of its prevalence in this specific setting
Schomerus and Hamster,[31] 2001	110	MHE	FPI	Impaired working abilities owing to MHE has a major impact on blue collar workers	The prevalence of MHE was not assessed by specific tests. Higher prevalence of alcoholic cirrhosis in blue collar workers
Marchesini et al,[15] 2001	554	Overt HE and MHE	SF-36, NHP	HE affects physical aspects more than mental aspects	Patients with HE failed to complete the questionnaires, with a high rate of missing data
Arguedas et al,[17] 2003	160	Overt HE and MHE	SF-36	Overt HE impairs both physical and mental aspects, whereas MHE mainly affects mental health	The test group is made of transplant candidates, who are expected to have a different prevalence of comorbidities and better social and health support
Bao et al,[36] 2007	106	MHE	SF-36, CLDQ	SF-36 scores are lower in patients with MHE, but no differences are shown in CLDQ scores	Sample includes patients with nonalcoholic cirrhosis and subjects who do not have cirrhosis (chronic hepatitis B)
Tan et al,[32] 2009	62 (36 at follow-up)	MHE	SIP	HRQoL remains significantly impaired at follow-up, after the resolution of MHE	Small sample of patients, many who were lost to follow-up
Wunsch et al,[33] 2011	77	MHE	SF-36, CLDQ	MHE does not significantly affect HRQoL in cirrhosis	Small sample of patients

Abbreviations: CLDQ, Chronic Liver Disease Questionnaire; FPI, Freiburg Personality Inventory; NHP, Nottingham Health Profile; SF-36, Medical Outcome Survey Short-Form 36; SIP, Sickness Impact Profile.

domains, with the notable exception of pain (**Fig. 1**).[15] Surprisingly, the physical components of health appeared to be more affected than the mental components of both inventories.[15] This unexpected finding is probably attributable to the poor insight that patients with HE have of their physical abilities.

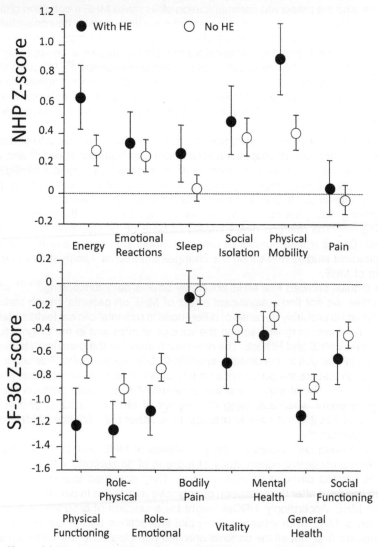

Fig. 1. Effect of hepatic encephalopathy on HRQoL in cirrhosis. Data were expressed as Z-scores, ie, as differences from normative values, adjusted for sex and age, on a scale having the standard deviation of the control population as unit of measure. Note that NHP scores are measures of distress, and positive values identify larger distress, whereas SF-36 scores are measures of HRQoL, and negative values identify poorer perceived health status. Also note that most scores were more severely affected in the presence of encephalopathy, with the notable exception of pain in both inventories, which was also not different from the normative population. (*Data from* Marchesini G, Bianchi G, Amodio P, et al. Factors associated with poor health-related quality of life of patients with cirrhosis. Gastroenterology 2001;120:170–8.)

Most studies linking poor HRQoL to HE have thus focused on the early form of HE, initially called subclinical, now defined as minimal hepatic encephalopathy (MHE), a mild cognitive impairment not detectable with a standard neurologic examination and not linked to sleep dysfunction or general problems with cognitive intelligence.[20–22] The absence of specific clinical manifestations, the lack of patients' insight into illness, and the preserved communication skills make MHE a condition difficult to diagnose.[23] The diagnosis should be performed with a careful neuropsychological examination, specific psychometric tests (or a standardized battery of tests, such as the Psychometric Hepatic Encephalopathy Score), and/or a neurophysiological assessment (electroencephalography, critical flicker frequency).[20] Although there is no *gold standard* method for detecting MHE, an early and correct diagnosis is important to avoid progression to overt HE (about 50% of untreated patients with MHE develop overt HE within 4–24 months),[24] with obvious negative consequences on HRQoL.[25]

The importance of MHE lies in its specific deficits, which are limited to certain abilities, such as attention, visuospatial abilities, and psychomotor speed,[26] and do not involve verbal and communication skills, with a preservation of global intelligence.[27] As any condition characterized by mild cognitive dysfunction, MHE may also have detrimental effects on HRQoL. In general, MHE implies a subclinical cognitive impairment involving mainly the most complex tasks, while preserving the basic activities of daily living.[28,29] The real and direct impact of MHE on HRQoL thus remains largely undefined. Only a limited number of cross-sectional studies are available, with very few longitudinal studies measuring the changes in patients' health status that follow the onset of MHE.

Some studies showed that MHE adversely affects daily functioning,[29–31] whereas other studies did not find a significant effect of MHE on patients' health status.[32,33] Such a debate is probably because of differences in patients' clinical features (etiology and severity of liver cirrhosis) among the various studies and in the diagnostic tools used to assess MHE and HRQoL. The most used tools are the generic questionnaires SF-36 and SIP, as well as the disease-specific CLDQ questionnaire. This last tool was developed to measure the burden of a variety of symptoms of liver disease, however, not merely MHE. The strong natural link between MHE and liver cirrhosis should be taken into account when assessing the impact of MHE on HRQoL, and in cross-sectional analyses it is not easy to distinguish whether the influence of MHE on QoL is true or spurious.[34]

Tan and colleagues[32] assessed the prevalence of MHE and its natural history in a short-term prospective cohort study of a group of 36 subjects with predominantly well-compensated cirrhosis of viral etiology. They observed that patients' HRQoL remained impaired after the resolution of cognitive alterations in patients initially diagnosed for MHE. Accordingly, HRQoL might be a function of progressive liver failure rather than of MHE, with influence on social interactions and emotions. This study has limitations: first, not all the patients enrolled participated in the follow-up evaluation; second, the diagnosis of MHE was based only on psychometric testing (at least one abnormal test); third, most patients had viral cirrhosis, and a viral etiology may be an independent cause of both impaired HRQoL and cognitive abilities, independent of liver failure and the presence of MHE.[35]

In a recent study on cirrhosis, the SF-36 and CLDQ scores were not significantly different between patients with and patients without MHE, diagnosed on the basis of Psychometric Hepatic Encephalopathy Score.[33] In this study, the relatively small number of subjects may have resulted in selection bias, reducing the validity of the results. In a larger study in a Chinese cohort,[36] no differences in CLDQ, except for abdominal symptoms, were confirmed in relation to the presence of MHE in patients with cirrhosis, whereas the scores of the SF-36 were lower in subjects with MHE. These results might be biased by the presence of a few patients who did not have cirrhosis (chronic hepatitis B). Moreover, the diagnosis of MHE was based on an abnormal slowing of the EEG and/or an abnormal score in at least one psychometric test (not as proposed by Ferenci and colleagues[20]), with the risk of overestimating MHE prevalence.

When the same diagnostic criteria were used in outpatients with a histologic diagnosis of liver cirrhosis,[29] no differences in SIP scores were demonstrated between patients with cirrhosis but without MHE and controls, whereas patients with MHE had a significant impairment in almost all domains, particularly in sleep and alertness, work, home management, and recreational activities. A multivariate analysis taking into account MHE, Child-Pugh score, presence of esophageal varices, and alcoholic etiology, only MHE appeared to be independently linked to a lower SIP score. A few years later, the same group tried to identify which of the domains explored by the SIP was most closely associated with MHE.[30] "I have difficulties doing handwork," "I am confused and start several actions at a time," and "I spent most of the day lying down to rest," all referring to daily functioning, were the statements most influenced by the presence of MHE. Moreover, the statement "I do not work at all" was strictly linked to MHE: up to 50% of patients with MHE had no permanent job, compared with 15% of those without MHE.

Impairment in working abilities could negatively affect HRQoL, because of the importance of a job as a component of personal satisfaction in Western countries; however, the mild cognitive alterations of MHE mainly involve practical intelligence and psychomotor functions, whereas global intelligence and verbal capabilities may be preserved.[37] Therefore, the specific cognitive dysfunction of MHE could have a different affect in different settings, for example between white collar workers (physicians, lawyers, managers) and blue collar workers (machinery operators, drivers, carpenters). Patients with cirrhosis engaged in professions that require sustained attention and motor coordination are more severely affected by MHE than those with jobs requiring predominantly verbal abilities.[31] In an outpatient cohort with liver cirrhosis, up to 60% of blue collar workers were considered unable to earn their living by the German social security system versus only 20% of white collar workers.[31] The study did not specifically assess the impact and prevalence of MHE in the 2 groups of workers, however. Most of the psychometric tests were similar in the 2 groups of patients, with the notable exclusion of tests measuring psychomotor functions (eg, fitness to driving), which were more significantly affected in nonworking patients. In general, blue collar workers also had a higher prevalence of alcoholic etiology, which might increase the prevalence of MHE.[38] Also in the presence of a similar MHE prevalence, the impact of cognitive dysfunction and impaired working ability remains larger in the blue collar group, where MHE interferes with complex occupational tasks and work performance, adversely affecting socioeconomic status,[39] with obvious consequences on QoL.

A sleep-wake pattern disruption is another early sign of HE[40]: insomnia, drowsiness, lethargy, and reversal of sleep rhythm are often the clinical presentation of overt HE and their presence and degree are used as an index for the severity of metabolic encephalopathy.[41] Sleep disturbances are also included as relevant items in the assessment of HRQoL in the NHP questionnaire, because of the importance of regular sleep in perceived health status. Patients with liver cirrhosis, regardless of the presence of HE, may experience sleep disorders that adversely affect their QoL,[42] but the correlation between sleep disturbances and cirrhosis or MHE is uncertain.

Montagnese and colleagues[43] assessed cognitive functions, quality of sleep, and HRQoL in 87 outpatients with biopsy-proven liver cirrhosis. They found no relationship between nighttime sleep disturbance and the presence or degree of HE; however, EEG slowing was more common in patients who reported a more pronounced daytime sleepiness, and the patients with more severe stages of HE were not able to complete the questionnaires. Thus, the authors cannot exclude a correlation between cognitive impairment and sleep abnormalities. These results are partly in keeping with seminal data on outpatients with liver cirrhosis, where no differences in the psychometric performance were found between subjects with or without sleep alterations.[44] Thus, cognitive abnormalities and sleep disturbances may be independent disorders that might both develop in patients with liver cirrhosis.

A link also exists between HRQoL and depression (**Box 1**), favoring social isolation, as well as anxiety/depression and sleep disorders. It might be argued that MHE, by interfering with patients' working abilities, daily functioning, and autonomy, might negatively affect patients' psychological status and lead to depression. Cognitive impairment and motor alterations might also synergistically lead to the onset of a depressed mood. Bianchi and colleagues[42] measured psychological status and depression in a group of 156 patients with cirrhosis, and did not find any correlation between sleep abnormalities and clinically detectable HE, but MHE was not investigated by appropriate tests. Mostacci and colleagues[45] showed that patients with MHE had more impaired sleep (daytime sleepiness and nighttime sleep disruption) than patients with cirrhosis without MHE. They also observed that a history of overt HE was not linked to alterations in sleep-wake patterns. A higher prevalence of insomnia and depression was also reported in patients with cirrhosis and early HE or MHE, compared with patients without any cognitive impairment.[46] The investigators proposed 2 hypotheses to support this evidence: (1) a somatic hypothesis, according to which the dysfunction of neurotransmitter systems involved in the pathogenesis of HE (in particular the serotoninergic system) might cause depression; and (2) a psychological hypothesis, according to which a deficit in coping strategies owing to HE might cause depression. During follow-up, however, they found that sleep disturbance and metabolic encephalopathy have an independent course. This implies that, although patients with MHE suffer from an important alteration of the circadian rhythm, the phenomenon may simply coexist with the cognitive impairment and is not its cause. Consequently, the disruption of the sleep-wake pattern cannot be used as a leading clinical symptom to diagnose HE or MHE.

There is growing evidence that psychological status and mood could not only interfere with disease history and response to treatment, but also adversely affect the outcome and morbidity/mortality in a wide range of medical conditions. Depression impairs social functioning, physical performance, and health status.[47] The presence

---

Box 1
Factors contributing to the relation between hepatic encephalopathy and poor HRQoL in cirrhosis

Severity of liver disease and complications

Cognitive dysfunction

Impaired motor skills

Depression

Sleep disorders

of sleep disturbance has a major impact on patients' psychological status, causing a higher prevalence of psychological disorders and depression. As suggested by Bianchi and colleagues,[42] the abnormalities in sleep-wake behavior could suggest the presence of an underlying psychiatric disorder or could themselves be involved in the pathogenesis of altered mood.

To summarize, abnormalities of the sleep-wake pattern and psychological status (mild depression, anxiety) are the most common psychopathological disorders in patients with cirrhosis, even if their correlation with HE and MHE is still unclear and discussed. Furthermore, at present there are no adequate tools able to distinguish the direct biologic impact of liver disease and HE on patients' psychopathological status from secondary psychological stressors owing to the chronic illness and its somatic manifestations.

EFFECTS OF TREATMENT ON HE AND HRQoL

Many different treatments have been proposed for MHE, on the basis of its pathogenesis linked to blood ammonia. A few treatments not only produced a reduction of cognitive impairment (which is the primary goal in the management of MHE), but also showed a significant improvement in HRQoL, confirming that cognitive dysfunction contributes to the poor perceived health status in patients with cirrhosis. Along this line, a positive effect of lactulose therapy on QoL had already been shown in some studies,[15] but only in recent years has there been a growing interest on the influence of drugs and other therapy on QoL. Prasad and colleagues[48] first specifically investigated the effect of treatment-related improvement in cognitive function on HRQoL. They enrolled 90 outpatients with cirrhosis but without a history of overt HE and found a greater impairment in patients with MHE compared with patients without MHE, mostly in psychosocial and physical subscores of the SIP inventory. At follow-up, patients with MHE treated with 3-month lactulose therapy showed a significant improvement of their HRQoL on several SIP subscores, particularly in emotional behavior, mobility, sleep/rest, and recreation and pastimes. Major limitations of this study were the absence of a placebo treatment arm and its nonblinded design.

Comparable results were reported following rifaximin treatment, a nonabsorbable antibiotic frequently prescribed to patients with MHE. In a pilot study involving 284 patients with cirrhosis,[49] 8 weeks of rifaximin therapy in patients with MHE significantly improved both neuropsychometric performance and SIP scores, confirming the strong relation between cognitive functions and QoL. In a multivariate analysis, MHE was significantly associated with the total SIP score. On the contrary, a 60-day probiotic yogurt supplementation had no effects on SF-36 scores in 25 patients with cirrhosis who were not alcoholic, but data could be affected by the small sample size, the low sensitivity of SF-36 in detecting subtle changes in QoL parameters, and the possible reduced effect of yogurt treatment compared with lactulose.[50] Similar data were observed following treatment with oral L-ornithine-L-aspartate[51] and acetyl-L-carnitine,[52] but more studies are needed.

SUMMARY

The initial symptoms of HE should be regarded as medical conditions significantly associated with poor perceived health status, and early diagnosis and treatment should be instituted to improve both cognitive impairment and HRQoL. The potential adverse effects of drug treatment for HE (diarrhea, bloating, and flatulence owing to lactulose and prebiotics) are of minor importance compared with the profound social isolation and impaired working abilities seen in advanced stages of the disease.

REFERENCES

1. The WHOQOL Group. Development of the World Health Organization WHOQOL-BREF quality of life assessment. Psychol Med 1998;28:551–8.
2. Aaronson NK. Quality of life: what is it? How should it be measured? Oncology 1998;2:69–76.
3. Spitzer WO. State of science 1986: quality of life and functional status as target variables for research. J Chronic Dis 1987;40:465–71.
4. Apolone G, De Carli G, Brunetti M, et al. Health-related quality of life (HR-QOL) and regulatory issues. An assessment of the European Agency for the Evaluation of Medicinal Products (EMEA) recommendations on the use of HR-QOL measures in drug approval. Pharmacoeconomics 2001;19:187–95.
5. Patrick DL, Deyo RA. Generic and disease-specific measures in assessing health status and quality of life. Med Care 1989;27:S217–32.
6. Guyatt GH, Juniper EF, Walter SD, et al. Interpreting treatment effects in randomised trials. BMJ 1998;316:690–3.
7. Lydick E, Epstein RS. Interpretation of quality of life changes. Qual Life Res 1993; 2(3):221–6.
8. Garratt A, Schmidt L, Mackintosh A, et al. Quality of life measurement: bibliographic study of patient assessed health outcome measures. BMJ 2002;324:1417.
9. Bergner M, Bobbitt RA, Carter WB, et al. The Sickness Impact Profile: development and final revision of a health status measure. Med Care 1981;19:787–805.
10. Hunt SM, McKenna SP, McEwen J, et al. A quantitative approach to perceived health status: a validation study. J Epidemiol Community Health 1980;34:281–6.
11. Hunt SM, McEwen J, McKenna SP. Measuring health status: a new tool for clinicians and epidemiologists. J R Coll Gen Pract 1985;35:185–8.
12. Ware JE Jr, Sherbourne CD. The MOS 36-item short-form health survey (SF-36). I. Conceptual framework and item selection. Med Care 1992;30:473–83.
13. Brazier JE, Harper R, Jones NM, et al. Validating the SF-36 health survey questionnaire: new outcome measure for primary care. BMJ 1992;305:160–4.
14. Younossi ZM, Guyatt G, Kiwi M, et al. Development of a disease specific questionnaire to measure health related quality of life in patients with chronic liver disease. Gut 1999;45:295–300.
15. Marchesini G, Bianchi G, Amodio P, et al. Factors associated with poor health-related quality of life of patients with cirrhosis. Gastroenterology 2001;120:170–8.
16. Younossi ZM, Boparai N, Price LL, et al. Health-related quality of life in chronic liver disease: the impact of type and severity of disease. Am J Gastroenterol 2001;96:2199–205.
17. Arguedas MR, DeLawrence TG, McGuire BM. Influence of hepatic encephalopathy on health-related quality of life in patients with cirrhosis. Dig Dis Sci 2003; 48:1622–6.
18. Martin LM, Sheridan MJ, Younossi ZM. The impact of liver disease on health-related quality of life: a review of the literature. Curr Gastroenterol Rep 2002;4: 79–83.
19. Ries ML, Jabbar BM, Schmitz TW, et al. Anosognosia in mild cognitive impairment: relationship to activation of cortical midline structures involved in self-appraisal. J Int Neuropsychol Soc 2007;13:450–61.
20. Ferenci P, Lockwood A, Mullen K, et al. Hepatic encephalopathy-definition, nomenclature, diagnosis, and quantification: final report of the working party at the 11th World Congresses of Gastroenterology, Vienna, 1998. Hepatology 2002;35:716–21.

21. Mullen KD. Review of the final report of the 1998 Working Party on definition, nomenclature and diagnosis of hepatic encephalopathy. Aliment Pharmacol Ther 2007;25(Suppl 1):11–6.
22. Ortiz M, Jacas C, Cordoba J. Minimal hepatic encephalopathy: diagnosis, clinical significance and recommendations. J Hepatol 2005;42(Suppl):S45–53.
23. Bajaj JS. Minimal hepatic encephalopathy matters in daily life. World J Gastroenterol 2008;14:3609–15.
24. Saxena N, Bhatia M, Joshi YK, et al. Electrophysiological and neuropsychological tests for the diagnosis of subclinical hepatic encephalopathy and prediction of overt encephalopathy. Liver 2002;22:190–7.
25. Davies MG, Rowan MJ, Feely J. EEG and event related potentials in hepatic encephalopathy. Metab Brain Dis 1991;6:175–86.
26. Amodio P, Del Piccolo F, Marchetti P, et al. Clinical features and survival of cirrhotic patients with subclinical cognitive alterations detected by the number connection test and computerized psychometric tests. Hepatology 1999;29:1662–7.
27. Weissenborn K, Ennen JC, Schomerus H, et al. Neuropsychological characterization of hepatic encephalopathy. J Hepatol 2001;34:768–73.
28. Dhiman RK, Chawla YK. Minimal hepatic encephalopathy. Indian J Gastroenterol 2009;28:5–16.
29. Groeneweg M, Quero JC, De Bruijn I, et al. Subclinical hepatic encephalopathy impairs daily functioning. Hepatology 1998;28:45–9.
30. Groeneweg M, Moerland W, Quero JC, et al. Screening of subclinical hepatic encephalopathy. J Hepatol 2000;32:748–53.
31. Schomerus H, Hamster W. Quality of life in cirrhotics with minimal hepatic encephalopathy. Metab Brain Dis 2001;16:37–41.
32. Tan HH, Lee GH, Thia KT, et al. Minimal hepatic encephalopathy runs a fluctuating course: results from a three-year prospective cohort follow-up study. Singapore Med J 2009;50:255–60.
33. Wunsch E, Szymanik B, Post M, et al. Minimal hepatic encephalopathy does not impair health-related quality of life in patients with cirrhosis: a prospective study. Liver Int 2011;31:980–4.
34. Amodio P. Health related quality of life and minimal hepatic encephalopathy. It is time to insert 'quality' in health care. J Gastroenterol Hepatol 2009;24:329–30.
35. Cordoba J, Flavia M, Jacas C, et al. Quality of life and cognitive function in hepatitis C at different stages of liver disease. J Hepatol 2003;39:231–8.
36. Bao ZJ, Qiu DK, Ma X, et al. Assessment of health-related quality of life in Chinese patients with minimal hepatic encephalopathy. World J Gastroenterol 2007;13:3003–8.
37. Schomerus H, Hamster W. Neuropsychological aspects of portal-systemic encephalopathy. Metab Brain Dis 1998;13:361–77.
38. Quero JC, Hartmann IJ, Meulstee J, et al. The diagnosis of subclinical hepatic encephalopathy in patients with cirrhosis using neuropsychological tests and automated electroencephalogram analysis. Hepatology 1996;24:556–60.
39. Stewart CA, Smith GE. Minimal hepatic encephalopathy. Nat Clin Pract Gastroenterol Hepatol 2007;4:677–85.
40. Martino ME, Romero-Vives M, Fernandez-Lorente J, et al. Sleep electroencephalogram alterations disclose initial stage of encephalopathy. Methods Find Exp Clin Pharmacol 2002;24(Suppl D):119–22.
41. Blei AT, Cordoba J. Hepatic encephalopathy. Am J Gastroenterol 2001;96:1968–76.

42. Bianchi G, Marchesini G, Nicolino F, et al. Psychological status and depression in patients with liver cirrhosis. Dig Liver Dis 2005;37:593–600.
43. Montagnese S, Middleton B, Skene DJ, et al. Night-time sleep disturbance does not correlate with neuropsychiatric impairment in patients with cirrhosis. Liver Int 2009;29:1372–82.
44. Cordoba J, Cabrera J, Lataif L, et al. High prevalence of sleep disturbance in cirrhosis. Hepatology 1998;27:339–45.
45. Mostacci B, Ferlisi M, Baldi Antognini A, et al. Sleep disturbance and daytime sleepiness in patients with cirrhosis: a case control study. Neurol Sci 2008;29: 237–40.
46. Wiltfang J, Nolte W, Weissenborn K, et al. Psychiatric aspects of portal-systemic encephalopathy. Metab Brain Dis 1998;13:379–89.
47. Wells KB, Stewart A, Hays RD, et al. The functioning and well-being of depressed patients. Results from the Medical Outcomes Study. JAMA 1989;262:914–9.
48. Prasad S, Dhiman RK, Duseja A, et al. Lactulose improves cognitive functions and health-related quality of life in patients with cirrhosis who have minimal hepatic encephalopathy. Hepatology 2007;45:549–59.
49. Sidhu SS, Goyal O, Mishra BP, et al. Rifaximin improves psychometric performance and health-related quality of life in patients with minimal hepatic encephalopathy (the RIME Trial). Am J Gastroenterol 2011;106:307–16.
50. Bajaj JS, Saeian K, Christensen KM, et al. Probiotic yogurt for the treatment of minimal hepatic encephalopathy. Am J Gastroenterol 2008;103:1707–15.
51. Ong JP, Oehler G, Kruger-Jansen C, et al. Oral L-ornithine-L-aspartate improves health-related quality of life in cirrhotic patients with hepatic encephalopathy: an open-label, prospective, multicentre observational study. Clin Drug Investig 2011;31:213–20.
52. Malaguarnera M, Bella R, Vacante M, et al. Acetyl-L-carnitine reduces depression and improves quality of life in patients with minimal hepatic encephalopathy. Scand J Gastroenterol 2011;46:750–9.

Index

Note: Page numbers of article titles are in **boldface** type.

A

Acarbose
  in fecal flora modulation
    in OHE management, 81–82
Activated charcoal
  ammonia reduction by
    in OHE management, 81
Adipopenia
  defined, 97
Adult fat malnutrition
  defined, 97
Aging
  cirrhosis effects of, 113
Amino acid imbalance
  false neurotransmitters and
    in HE pathogenesis, 11
γ-Aminobutyric acid (GABA)
  ammonia and brain extracellular concentrations of
    in HE pathogenesis, 19
γ-Aminobutyric acid (GABA)–mediated inhibitory neurotransmission
  in HE pathogenesis, 11–16
γ-Aminobutyric acid (GABA) receptor
  ammonia effects on, 17
γ-Aminobutyric acid (GABA) receptor complex
  synergistic interaction between ammonia and agonist ligands of, 17–19
Ammonia
  neurosteroids and
    in HE pathogenesis, 19
  reduction of
    nonabsorbable disaccharides in
      in OHE management, 79–81
Ammonia hypothesis
  in HE pathogenesis, 9–10, 16–19
    ammonia and brain extracellular concentration of GABA, 19
    ammonia and neurosteroids, 19
    ammonia effects on $GABA_A$ receptor, 17
    significance of ammonia concentrations in, 17
    synergistic interaction between ammonia and agonist ligands of $GABA_A$ receptor
      complex, 17–19
    variants of, 10

Clin Liver Dis 16 (2012) 171–181
doi:10.1016/S1089-3261(12)00011-6
1089-3261/12/$ – see front matter © 2012 Elsevier Inc. All rights reserved.

liver.theclinics.com

Moving?

Make sure your subscription moves with you!

To notify us of your new address, find your **Clinics Account Number** (located on your mailing label above your name), and contact customer service at:

Email: journalscustomerservice-usa@elsevier.com

800-654-2452 (subscribers in the U.S. & Canada)
314-447-8871 (subscribers outside of the U.S. & Canada)

Fax number: 314-447-8029

Elsevier Health Sciences Division
Subscription Customer Service
3251 Riverport Lane
Maryland Heights, MO 63043

*To ensure uninterrupted delivery of your subscription, please notify us at least 4 weeks in advance of move.

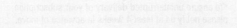

Printed and bound by CPI Group (UK) Ltd, Croydon, CR0 4YY

03/10/2024

01040449-0016